RESTRICTED GROWTH - CLINICAL, GENETIC AND MOLECULAR ASPECTS

Edited by **María del Carmen Cárdenas-Aguayo**

Restricted Growth - Clinical, Genetic and Molecular Aspects
http://dx.doi.org/10.5772/61620
Edited by María del Carmen Cárdenas-Aguayo

Contributors

Mauro Bozzola, Cristina Meazza, Monica Mottes, Patricia Marie Jeanne Lievens, Diana Miclea, Leandro Fernández-Pérez, Diego Iglesias-Gato, Amilcar Flores-Morales, Juan Carlos Díaz-Chico, Carlos Borja Guerra-Hernández, stefano stagi, Annachiara Azzali, Luisa La Spina, Matteo Della Monica, Perla Scalini, Maurizio De Martino, Guy-Joseph Lemamy

Published by InTech

Janeza Trdine 9, 51000 Rijeka, Croatia

Publishing Process Manager Edi Lipovic

Technical Editor SPi Global

Cover InTech Design team

First published October, 2016

Printed in Croatia

Additional hard copies can be obtained from orders@intechopen.com

Restricted Growth - Clinical, Genetic and Molecular Aspects, Edited by María del Carmen Cárdenas-Aguayo

p. cm.

Print ISBN 978-953-51-2694-2
Online ISBN 978-953-51-2695-9

For EU product safety concerns:
IN TECH d.o.o., Prolaz Marije Krucifikse Kozulić 3, 51000 Rijeka, Croatia,
info@intechopen.com or visit our website at intechopen.com.

Meet the editor

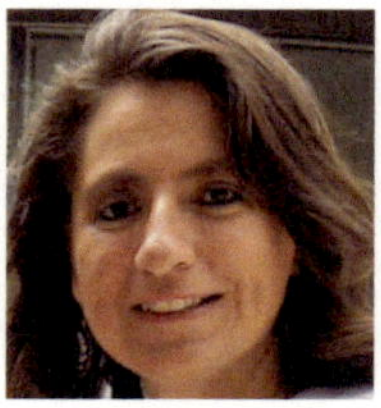

Maria del Carmen Cárdenas-Aguayo, PhD, is currently a Professor in the Department of Physiology, School of Medicine, Universidad Nacional Autónoma de México (UNAM), Mexico City, Mexico. Her laboratory engages in multidisciplinary research to elucidate the molecular mechanisms of neuronal differentiation and the study of the effects of cellular stress and protein recycling impairments on neurodegeneration. Her research has been directed at studying the differentiation potential of hippocampal neural precursor cells from mouse and human models and its implication in neurological disorders. Her studies in molecular medicine started during her MS thesis work at CINVESTAV-IPN, Mexico City, Mexico, and continued with her PhD in molecular biomedicine on the neurosciences field at CINVESTAV-IPN, Mexico City, Mexico. Subsequently, she accomplished two international research trainings, one at the Nathan Kline Institute, Center for Dementia Research, Orangeburg, NY, and the other at the Institute for Basic Research in Developmental Disabilities, Staten Island, NY. Prior to her arrival at the School of Medicine, UNAM, Dr. Cárdenas-Aguayo held a Visiting Professor position at CINVESTAV-IPN, Mexico City, Mexico.

Contents

Preface

Restricted growth conditions are a group of genetic disorders with primary effect on growth (short stature); it is very heterogeneous and comprises two important categories: skeletal dysplasia and different genetic syndromes with primary effect on growth. It could also be caused by a medical condition. Their diagnosis is often difficult, but it is essential to get it early in the life of the affected individuals, in order to give the appropriate treatment that could restore at least partially the growth allowing the subject to reach the closest to the average height as possible in adulthood.

The book discusses the genetic mutations associated to restricted growth (dwarfism phenotype), at the clinical, cellular, and molecular levels, and comparisons among phenotypes.

There are several different types of dwarfism; some of them are caused by mutations on the FGF3R. It is known that this pathway, FGF3R signaling, negatively regulates bone growth. In this book, the importance of this pathway on bone growth regulation and dwarfism is discussed.

The book contains chapters regarding different aspects of the study of restricted growth that are divided into three broad sections:

Section I: Defining Restricted Growth (Chapter 1: Growth Hormone Axis in Skeletal Dysplasias)

Section II: Genetics and Diagnosis of Restricted Growth (Chapter 2: Growth Hormone Deficiency: Diagnosis and Therapy in Children and Chapter 3: Genetic Determinants of Short Stature)

Section III: Signaling Pathways and Molecular Mechanisms of Restricted Growth (Chapter 4: Molecular Defects and Cellular Dysfunctions in Restricted Growth Conditions, Chapter 5: Growth Hormone Receptor Signaling Pathways and Its Negative Regulation by SOCS2, and Chapter 6: Mannose-6-Phosphate/Insulin-Like Growth Factor 2 Receptor (M6P/IGF2R) in Growth and Disease: A Review)

The book presents comprehensive reviews of each topic written by experts in the field. This book will be the most valuable tool for physicians and life science researchers as well as contribute in the training of biomedical students. We hope that this book will motivate more discussion and research in this important health problem that would set the path for finding better therapeutic approaches for these groups of restricted growth disorders.

Section I: Defining Restricted Growth, starts with Chapter 1: Growth Hormone Axis in Skeletal Dysplasias by Stagi et al., it introduces the reader to the main common skeletal dysplasias, such as achondroplasia, hypochondroplasia, 3M syndrome, and Leri-Weill syndrome;

providing the clinical, radiological, and genetic aspects of these restricted growth conditions that allow their classification; and provide a discussion of the data available about growth, final height (FH), height velocity (HV), growth hormone deficiency, and growth hormone response after growth hormone (GH) treatment in patients with skeletal dysplasias.

Section II: Genetics and Diagnosis of Restricted Growth, starts with Chapter 2: Growth Hormone Deficiency: Diagnosis and Therapy in Children. Bozzola and Meazza discussed the growth hormone deficiency (GHD) associated with restricted growth in children, adolescents, and young adults. Pituitary hormone deficiencies (combined pituitary hormone deficiency (CPHD)) associated with GHD are also discussed. This chapter talks about genetics of GHD and the diagnostic strategies and protocols for diagnosis and the efficacy of the rhGH therapy. Interestingly, this chapter addresses the issue of GH treatment of children after bone marrow transplantation (BMT) for acute leukemia, which is another application of the rhGH therapy that has to be taken into account due to the increased incidence of cancer in children and the impact of chemotherapy and radiation on children's growth rate.

Chapter 3 of Section II: Genetic Determinants of Short Stature, by Miclea, provides a comprehensive discussion of the group of genetic disorders that affect growth, which is very heterogeneous. The chapter talks about the main classification of these disorders in skeletal dysplasia and the different genetic syndromes with primary effect on growth. And the main clinical signs of each syndrome are discussed and an algorithm for clinical diagnosis and genetic testing that is a very useful tool for clinical and etiologic diagnosis is provided.

Section III: Signaling Pathways and Molecular Mechanisms of Restricted Growth, begins with Chapter 4: Molecular Defects and Cellular Dysfunctions in Restricted Growth Conditions by Mottes and Lievens, in which selected conditions associated with restricted growth are addressed. In particular, classifications, phenotypical characteristics, and cellular and molecular aspects are discussed. The genetic classification is given according to the Online Mendelian Inheritance in Man (OMIM), which is useful for the geneticists and physicians. Additionally, methods used in the studies discussed in the chapter are well described, which are useful to undergraduate and graduate students.

Chapter 5 of Section III: Growth Hormone Receptor Signaling Pathways and Its Negative Regulation by SOCS2, by Fernandez-Perez et al., provides a comprehensive discussion of the central role of GHR signaling in somatic growth regulation and the critical role of SOCS2 as a negative regulator of body growth. The role of SOCS2 in lipid metabolism and insulin signaling is also discussed. This chapter makes reference to the potential therapeutic applications of targeting SOCS2-regulated pathways. It talks about the complex steroid interactions with GHR signaling in physiological (sex determination and somatic growth) and pathological states (dwarfism and sexual dimorphism). The role of SOCS2 as ubiquitin ligase in promoting ubiquitination of GHR and its subsequent degradation by the proteasome, contributing to the termination of the GH intracellular signaling, is also addressed.

Chapter 6 of Section III: Mannose-6-Phosphate/Insulin-Like Growth Factor 2 Receptor (M6P/IGF2R) in Growth and Disease: A Review, by Lemamy et al., is the final part of the last section of this book, in which the authors review the role of M6P/IGF2R in the regulation of growth and development and its involvement in tumor progression. Interestingly, this chapter talks about the involvement of M6P/IGF2R in the trafficking of mannose-6-phosphorylated enzymes from the trans-Golgi network (TGN) to lysosomes and the uptake of secreted proenzymes from the plasma membrane to the lysosomes via clathrin-coated vesicles for their maturation. Therefore, this chapter mentions that the M6P/IGF2R acts as a scavenger that binds IGF2 and transports it to lysosomes for its degradation. Consequently, M6P/IGF2R is considered as a scavenger that regulates IGF2 levels before it reaches IGF1 receptor to exert its biological effects on cell proliferation and growth. In this chapter, the fact that there is a reduction in the expression of M6P/IGF2R in cancer cells as compared to normal cells in about 50% of breast tumors, which led to suggest its potential value as a cancer prognostic marker, is also discussed.

Finally, this chapter highlights that insulin-like growth factor axis has a critical role in mediating fetal and postnatal growth; thus, alterations in this pathway including changes in the expression of the M6P/IGF2 receptor and impairments in its function could impact somatic growth. Moreover, genetic evidence clearly supports a role for IGF2/M6P receptors in organ development and growth.

I am grateful to InTech— Open Access Publisher for initiating this book project and for asking me to serve as its editor. I want to thank Mr. Edi Lipović, Publishing Process Manager, and Ana Pantar, Senior Commissioning Editor, at InTech for guiding me through the publication process and coordinating the different steps involved. I also want to thank all the contributors of this book for writing their chapters, for sharing their knowledge of the field, and for making my requested revisions to them. I am grateful to all editorial team of InTech, for their efforts in facilitating the access of knowledge to many researches worldwide through its open access publications. I would like to thank my family (especially my mother, Montessori Guide Carmen Aguayo-Briz), for their support and comprehension during this book project and throughout my scientific career.

María del Carmen Cárdenas-Aguayo, PhD
Professor
Department of Physiology, School of Medicine
Universidad Nacional Autónoma de México (UNAM)
Mexico City, Mexico

Section 1

Defining Restricted Growth

Chapter 1

Growth Hormone Axis in Skeletal Dysplasias

Stefano Stagi, Annachiara Azzali, Luisa La Spina,
Matteo Della Monica, Perla Scalini and
Maurizio de Martino

Additional information is available at the end of the chapter

http://dx.doi.org/10.5772/64802

Abstract

Introduction: Skeletal dysplasias, also termed as osteochondrodysplasias, are a large heterogeneous group of disorders characterized by abnormalities of bone or cartilage growth or texture. They occur due to genetic mutations and their phenotype continues to evolve throughout life. Reduced growth is a common feature.

Objective: To evaluate and discuss data about growth and growth hormone axis in patients with the main common skeletal dysplasias, such as achondroplasia, hypochondroplasia, 3M syndrome, and Leri-Weill syndrome.

Design: Evaluate retrospectively the data on growth, final height (FH), height velocity (HV), growth hormone deficiency, and growth hormone response after growth hormone (GH) treatment in patients with these disorders. However, this chapter provides an updated picture of growth hormone axis and endocrinological features in skeletal dysplasia.

Keywords: growth, growth hormone, skeletal dysplasia

1. Introduction

Skeletal dysplasias are a genetically and clinically heterogeneous group of disorders associated with generalized abnormalities in the skeleton. Collectively the birth incidence is estimated to be about 1:5000 live births [1], but it is probably underestimated due to the large amount of undiagnosed cases. The most evident clinical aspects are the skeletal abnormalities, which can anyway be associated to orthopaedic, neurologic, auditory, visual, pulmonary, cardiac, renal and psychological complications. The clinical expression of these pathologies can range from a precocious arthropathy in otherwise healthy individuals to severe dwarfism with perinatal mortality [2].

Many different types of dysplasias have been described and classified depending on the clinical, radiological and genetic aspects. In the latest 2015 version of nosology, compared to the one of 2011, the overall number has decreased to 436 disorders, but the number of groups has increased to 42 and the number of genes to 364 [3] (**Table 1**).

Type	Composition	Distribution	Pathology	Gene	Location
I	$\alpha1[I]_2\alpha2[I]$	Dermis, bone, tendon, ligament	Osteogenesis imperfecta (OI) I, II, III, IV, VIIA. Ehler-Danlos syndrome (EDS) classic	*COL1A1, OI1, OI2, OI3, OI4, EDSC*	17q21.33
			OI II, OI III, OI IV, OI VIIB, EDS (valvular form), osteoporosis	*COL1A2*	7q21.3
II	$\alpha1[II]_3$	Cartilage, vitreous	Otospondylomegaepiphyseal dysplasia, spondyloperipheral dysplasia, osteoarthritis with mild chondrodysplasia, spondyloe-piphyseal dysplasia, Stanescu type, achondrogenesis, type II or hypochondrogenesis, SMED Strudwick type, vitreoretinopathy with phalangeal epiphyseal dysplasia, Kniest dysplasia, SED congenita, Stickler syndrome, type I, epiphyseal dysplasia, multiple, with myopia and deafness, platyspondylic skeletal dysplasia, Torrance type, stickler syndrome, type I, nonsyndromic ocular, Czech ?? dysplasia	*COL2A1*	12q13.11
III	$\alpha1[III]_3$	Skin, blood vessels, intestine	Ehler-Danlos syndrome type IV	*COL3A1*	2q32.2
IV	$\alpha1[IV]_2\alpha2[IV]$ $\alpha3[IV]$ $\alpha4[IV]$ $\alpha5[IV]$ $\alpha5[IV]$, $\alpha6[IV]$	Basement membranes	Susceptibility to intracerebral, haemorrhage, porencephaly, brain small vessel disease with or without ocular anomalies, angiopathy, hereditary, with nephropathy, aneurysms, and muscle cramps Susceptibility to intracerebral haemorrhage, porencephaly	*COL4A1,POREN1,* *HANAC, ICH, BSVD* *COL4A2, POREN2,* *ICH* *COL4A3* *COL4A4* *COL4A5, ATS, ASLN*	13q34 13q34 2q36.3 2q36.3 Xq22.3

http://dx.doi.org/10.5772/64802

Type	Composition	Distribution	Pathology	Gene	Location
			Alport syndrome (autosomal recessive and autosomal dominant), familial benign haematuria Alport syndrome, familial benign haematuria Alport syndrome		
V	α1[V]$_3$ α1[V]$_2$α2[V] α1[V] α2[V] α3[V]	Bone, dermis, cornea, placenta	Ehler-Danlos syndrome (classic type) Ehler-Danlos syndrome (classic type) –	*COL5A1, EDSC* *COL5A2, EDSC* *COL5A3*	9q34.3 2q32.2 19p13.2
VI	α1[VI] α2[VI] α3[VI] α1[VI] α2[VI] α4[VI]	Bone, dermis, cornea, cartilage	Bethlem myopathy, Ullrich congenital muscular dystrophy 1 Bethlem myopathy, Ullrich congenital muscular dystrophy 1 Bethlem myopathy, Ullrich congenital muscular dystrophy 1, segmental isolated dystonia – – –	*COL6A1, BTHLM1, UCHMD1* *COL6A2, BTHLM1, UCMD1* *COL6A3,, DYT27, BTHLM1, UCMD1* *COL6A4* *COL6A5, COL29A1* *COL6A6*	21q22.3 21q22.3 2q37.3 3q22.1, 3p25.1 3q22.1 3q22.1
VII	α1[VII]$_2$ α2[VII]	Dermis, bladder	Epidermolysis bullosa, Isolated toenail dystrophy	*COL7A1, NDNC8*	3p21.31
VIII	α1[VIII]$_3$ α2[VIII]$_3$ α1[VIII]$_2$ α2[VIII]	Dermis, brain, heart, kidney	– Corneal dystrophy	*COL8A1* *COL8A2, FECD1, PPCD2*	3q12.1 1p34.3
IX	α1[IX] α2[IX] α3[IX]	Cartilage, cornea, vitreous	Stickler syndrome type IV, multiple epiphyseal dysplasia Stickler syndrome type V, multiple epiphyseal dysplasia Multiple epiphyseal dysplasia with miopathy, multiple epiphyseal dysplasia	*COL9A1, EDM6, STL4COL9A2, EDM2, STL5COL9A3, EDM3, IDD*	6q13 1p34.2 20q13.33
X	α1[X]$_3$	Cartilage	Metaphyseal chondrodysplasia type Schmid	*COL10A1*	6q22.1
XI	α1[XI] α2[XI] α3[XI]	Cartilage, intervertebral disc	Marshall syndrome, fibrochondrogenesis, Stickler syndrome type II Deafness, Weissenbacher-Zweymuller syndrome, Stickler syndrome type III,	*COL11A1, STL2* *COL11A2, STL3, DFNA13, DFNB53, FBCG2*	1p21.1 6p21.32

Type	Composition	Distribution	Pathology	Gene	Location
			otospondylomegaepiphyseal dysplasia, fibrochondrogenesis		
XII	$\alpha1[XII]_3$	Dermis, tendon	Bethlem myopathy 2, Ullrich congenital muscular dystrophy 2	*COL12A1, UCMD2, BTHLM2*	6q13-q14
XIII	–	Endothelial cells, dermis, eye, heart	Congenital myasthenic syndrome	*COL13A1*	10q22.1
XIV	$\alpha1[XIV]_3$	Bone, dermis, cartilage	–	*COL14A1, UND*	8q24.12
XV	–	Capillaris, testis, kidney, heart	–	*COL15A1*	9q22.33
XVI	–	Dermis, kidney	–	*COL16A1*	1p35.2
XVII	–	Hemidesmosomes in epithelia	Generalized atrophic epidermolysis bullosa	*COL17A1, BPAG2, ERED*	10q25.1
XVIII	–	Basement membrane, liver	Knobloch syndrome	*COL18A1, KNO1*	21q22.3
XIX	–	basement membrane	–	*COL19A1, D6S228E, COL9A1L*	6q13
XX	–	Cornea	–	–	–
XXI	–	Stomach, kidney	–	*COL21A1*	6p12.1
XXII	–	Heart, retina	–	*COL22A1*	8q24.2–q24.3
XXIII	–	Brain, cornea	–	*COL23A1*	5q35.3
XXIV	–	Bone, cornea	–	*COL24A1*	1p22.3
XXV	–	Brain, heart, testis	Amyloid formation, Congenital fibrosis of extraocular muscles	*COL25A1, CLAC, CFEOM5*	4q25
XXVI	–	Testis, ovary	–	*SH2B1, SH2B, KIAA1299*	7q22.1
XXVII	–	Cartilage	Steel syndrome	*COL27A1, KIAA1870, STLS*	9q32
XXVIII	–	Dermis, sciatic nerve	Neurodegenerative disease	*COL28A1*	7p21.3

Table 1. Main common skeletal dysplasias.

2. Physiology

The human skeleton is a complex organ composed of 206 bones (126 appendicular, 74 axial and 6 ossicles). It strictly collaborates with the muscle, tendons and cartilages in order allow

http://dx.doi.org/10.5772/64802

movement, mechanical support, linear growth and to protect internal organs. The bone is also involved in the calcium phosphorus metabolism and in the haematopoiesis.

The skeletal system develops from mesoderm. The mesodermal cells form the mesenchyme (embryonic connective tissue), which can differentiate into fibroblasts, chondroblasts, and osteoblasts. Initially, the mesenchyme appears uncondensed, then the cells come together to the sites of future bones and joints. How does it occur? Two mechanisms are involved, depending on the cell differentiation into osteoblasts or chondrocyte: there will be respectively a membranous or an endochondral ossification. The first one occurs especially in the calvaria of the skull, the maxilla, the mandible and in the subperiosteal bone, forming layer of long bones. The osteoblasts produce an extracellular matrix, called osteoid. Those of them which remain incorporated into the osteoid become osteocytes. Finally, the osteoid becomes mineralized, thus forming the mature bone tissue.

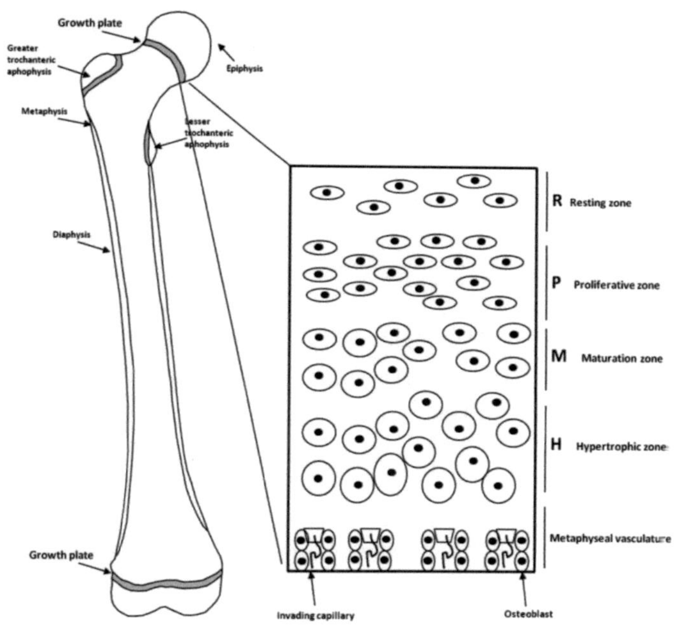

Figure 1. Anatomical representation of the femoral growth plate.

The endochondral ossification represents the mayor mechanism of formation of most of the mammalian appendicular skeleton. The first site of ossification is in the middle of the diaphysis, while the second one occurs in the epiphysis. They start from a differentiation of mesenchymal cells into chondrocytes, forming the cartilage model, which in turn, undergoes a process of proliferation, hypertrophy and degradation. Through the periosteal buds, osteoclasts (that remove the cartilage extracellular matrix (ECM)), osteoblasts (that deposit bone on cartilage remnants) and blood vessels invade the model and proceed to form the primary centre of ossification. In long bones, a secondary centre of ossification formed at each end of the cartilage model. The cartilaginous growth plate that remains between the two ossification centres allows the linear growth until the postpubertal age, when it will be completely replaced by bone [4] (**Figure 1**). Finally, there is an appositional growth due to the periosteum's osteoblasts, leading to the formation of a bone collar that works as support for the new bone [5].

The growth plate, depending on the stage of cell's maturation, can be divided in the following zones (**Figure 1**) [6]

- The resting/germinative zone, in which the stem cells or progenitor cells continuously replace the pool of proliferative chondrocytes.
- The proliferative zone, where highly proliferating chondrocytes are disposed into column parallel to the direction of longitudinal growth and produces ECM.
- The pre-hypertrophic zone, where chondrocytes initiate the hypertrophic differentiation, characterized by IHH (Indian Hedgehog) expression (see below).
- The hypertrophic zone is constituted by enlarged chondrocytes that increase in length, thus determining the bone's lengthening; they also modify the surrounding ECM mineralizing it.
- The degeneration zone, where chondrocytes undergo rapid death before ossification.

Chondrocytes are involved in the production of the ECM, which is majorly composed by collagen. Collagens are single molecules composed by amino acid sequence of glycine-proline-X and glycine-X-hydroxyproline, where X is any amino acid other than glycine, proline or hydroxyproline. These amino acids associate into chains to form a triple helical structure. Once in the extracellular matrix, the triple helical chain undergoes several biochemical and structural modifications, becoming a fibril. The collagen family comprises 28 members that contain at least one triple-helical domain [7] and that are specifically distributed in different parts of the body. Collagens are classified in fibrillar types (I, II, III, V and XI) and non-fibrillar, depending on the structure they form in the extracellular matrix. Type I is the most expressed in the human body and with the other collagens provide mechanical strength of cartilage, bone and skin [2, 7]. Other widely represented collagens are type II (hyaline cartilage) and IV (in the basal membrane). if a mutation occurs in any of the genes encoding collagens molecules, a skeletal dysplasia can be developed.

3. Growth plate and hormones

The growth plate maturation and regulation is influenced by growth factors, local regulators and hormones (**Figure 2**). Perichondrial cells produce many different growth factors that are used as a signal to chondrocytes, but they also receive signals back from epiphyseal cells (**Figure 2**). An important role in bone formation is played by parathyroid hormone-related protein (PTHrP) and Ihh; they act directly on the differentiation and proliferation of chondrocytes and in the differentiation of osteoblast. The paracrine hormone PTHrP is expressed at high level in early proliferating chondrocytes at the end of long bones, while its receptor Pthr1 is produced at low levels by proliferating growth plate chondrocytes and at higher level in prehypertrophic cells [8]. Prehypertrophic and hypertrophic chondrocytes secrete Ihh, a member of the hedegehog family, which acts through the binding to receptor Patched-1 [9]. PTHrP and Ihh are connected in a feedback loop to maintain a pool of immature chondrocyte progenitors. PTHrP acts on the receptor of chondrocyte to keep them proliferating and delays the differentiation into pre-hypertrophic and hypertrophic chondrocytes. Once the cells are too far from the source of PTHrP production, in the transitional zone between proliferating and hypertrophic chondrocytes, Ihh begins to be secreted. It increases the proliferation rate and inhibits terminal differentiation of chondrocytes; moreover, it stimulates PTHrP synthesis [10]. Mutations in these two genes can cause the development of dysplasias, as for example the acrocapitofemoral dysplasia is associated with a Ihh mutation [11]. Bone morphogenetic proteins (BMPs) signal contribute to epiphyseal growth and maturation, thanks to a gradient of proteins expressed in the growth plate: BMP agonists can be found in the hypertrophic zone, while BMP antagonists in the resting zone, suggesting a role in the spatial regulation [12]. Fibroblast growth factor (FGF) signalling interact both with BMP and Ihh pathways, inhibiting chondrocyte proliferation. In fact, FGF act as antagonists of BMP signalling and negatively regulate Ihh expression, thus controlling the process of hypertrophic differentiation to the proliferation rate [13]. The role of FGF signalling is clearly demonstrated in achondroplasia, which is due to a mutation in FGF3 (fibroblast growth factor 3) receptor. Wnt signalling is then involved in chondrocytes development, differentiation and in the osteoblasts formation. The Runt family transcription factor Runx2 (runt-related transcription factor 2) and Runx3 contribute to chondrocyte hypertrophy and co-operate with TGF-β in the regulation of their maturation. TGF-β actually acts at the beginning as a stimulator of chondrocyte's differentiation, stabilizing than the epiphyseal chondrocyte in a prehypertrophic stage (**Figure 2**) [14].

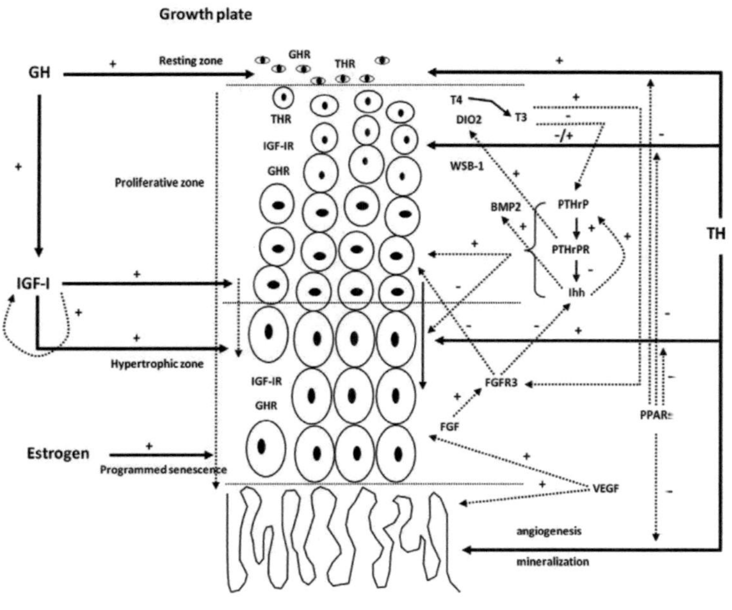

Figure 2. Main hormonal and non-hormonal actions on the growth plate. Modified by Seminara et al. [16].

Finally, the vascular endothelial growth factor seems to play a role in the epiphyseal fusion, stimulating the chondrocyte differentiation, chondrocyte survival, and the final stages of endochondral ossification. It seems to be active especially during puberty, under the stimulus of oestrogens [15]; anyway, the role it plays in oestrogen-mediated growth plate remains elusive (**Figure 2**).

As previously reported, not only growth factors but also hormones can influence bone growth. It is commonly known that sexual hormones are involved in the regulation of skeletal growth and in its maintenance. Oestrogens, especially 17β-estradiol (E2), act via the oestrogen receptor-a (ER-a); low E2 levels during sexual maturation contribute to the lengthening of the bone during the growth spurt, while high levels in the late puberty to the growth plate closure. The mechanism by which oestrogen influence bones' growth is not yet clearly understood. As oestrogens can regulate also the growth hormone-insulin growth factor-1 (GH)/IGF-1) axis, the modulation of that pathway is able to condition bone maturation: low levels of E2 increase serum GH and IGF1, enhancing the pubertal spurt [17]. Sexual hormones are mainly produced by gonads, but they can be synthetized directly in the growth plate by the aromatase or other enzymes (17β hydroxysteroid dehydrogenase, steroid sulphatase and type 1 5-α reductase) produced by the chondrocytes (**Figure 2**) [11].

Androgen stimulates bone formation linking to androgen receptor (AR) directly or as dihydrotestosterone (DHT), as well as to ER following aromatization in estradiol [18]. AR is expressed by chondrocytes and regulate their proliferation and differentiation. An increment in growth plate width after injection of testosterone directly into the growth plate of rats, support the idea that it could have a direct function. It is not well known the effect of testosterone on osteoblast cell and controversial result have been shown, anyway most *in vitro* studies indicate that androgens contribute to osteoblast progenitors proliferation, mature osteoblast differentiation and osteoblasts apoptosis inhibition (**Figure 2**) [19].

Thyroid hormones play a role in bones' growth through an action both on chondrocytes and osteoblasts. Reserve and proliferating chondrocyte in fact express thyroid hormone receptor a1 (TRa1) and TRb1, indicating that T_3 contributes directly to the epiphyseals' growth. Experiments showed that T_3 inhibits chondrocyte clonal expansion and proliferation, while stimulating chondrocyte differentiation, suggesting a role in the regulation of bone formation [20].

Studies about T_3 action on osteoblast are contradictory; anyway, it is undoubted that it contributes to stimulate osteoblast activity. In fact, T_3 promotes type I collagen synthesis and posttranscriptional modification, induces alkaline phosphatase (involved in matrix mineralization), regulates synthesis and secretion of the bone matrix proteins osteopontin and osteocalcin; it is also involved in bone remodelling enhancing the production of matrix metallopeptidase 9 (MMP-9) and -13. Furthermore, T_3 regulates IGF-1 and FGF pathways. Moreover, through the regulation of osteoprotegerine levels, T_3 can influence bone resorption (**Figure 2**) [21].

Glucocorticoids are strictly involved in growth plate regulation. Increased levels of glucocorticoids determine an inhibition of longitudinal bone's growth. It has been demonstrated that glucocorticoids can inhibit chondrocyte proliferation, hypertrophy and cartilage matrix secretion. Glucocorticoids can affect bone also through their negative effect on muscle, influencing the normal modelling process [22]. Furthermore, glucocorticoids also slow growth plate senescence inhibiting the proliferation of the resting zone. This explains the catch up growth measured after a period of growth inhibition due to glucocorticoids excess. Once the inhibiting stimulus has been removed, the growth plates behave as "younger" growth plates, reaching the final height a bit later and more rapidly [23]. Last but not least is the role of GH and somatomedinic hormones, which will be discussed further (**Figure 2**).

4. Clinical manifestations

The main characteristic of the skeletal dysplasia is a disharmonic short stature; anyway, many other manifestations involving other organs have been described. How to recognize a dysplastic child? At first, the most important step is to examine the body proportions. Sometimes subtle degrees of the pathology could be difficult to appreciate, especially in obese or premature child.

In every child, it is essential to evaluate growth parameters such as height, weight and head circumference, but in skeletal dysplasias, these are not sufficient; it is in fact necessary to evaluate also sitting height, upper/lower segment ratio and arm span [1].

The sitting height is the distance from the vertex of the head to the surface where the child person is sitting erectly; it is used to measure the upper segment of the body. The lower segment can be calculated by subtracting the upper segment from the total height. With these parameters, it is possible to obtain the cormic index, which is the upper/lower ratio. The values of cormic index modify with age. It is important to remember that a patient with a short trunk has a decreased upper/lower segment ratio, while a short statured patient with normal trunk and relatively short limbs may have an increased upper/lower segment ratio [1]. Short trunk child could present short neck or small chest or protuberant abdomen. Depending on which part of the limb is involved, short limb dysplasias can be differentiated into three groups: rhizomelic shortening if proximal segments are involved (humerus and femur); mesomelic shortening if middle segments (radius, ulna, tibia and fibula) are involved; acromelic shortening involves distal segments as the hands and feet.

Finally, the spam arm measures the length from one fingertips to the other when arm raised parallel to the ground at shoulder height at 180° angle.

A general physical examination should always be made to detach others sign and dysmorphisms, which are useful to differentiate between numerous dysplasias. For example, the clavicular agenesis is typical of cleido-cranial dysplasia, or the blue sclera of osteogenesis imperfecta. Also facial dysmorphism can be pathognomonic: in the achondroplastic phenotype are present macrocephaly, frontal bossing, midface hypoplasia and short upturned noses; midface hypoplasia with flat nasal bridge and grey iris colour in the acrodysostosis; odonto-chodrodysplasia is characterized by dentinogenesis imperfecta.

It's also important to evaluate the child during the time and repeat the physical examination to notice other manifestation involving or the skeleton, like abnormal joint mobility or angular deformities (that usually are symmetric), or other organs, depending on the role of the gene involved.

Finally, it is essential to pay serious attention to major problems associated with skeletal dysplasia; for example, there is an increased risk to develop pneumonia due to a reduced pulmonary volume secondary to the short ribs or spinal cord compression at the cervical medullar junction due to an abnormal growth of the base of the skull and the vertebral pedicles. In Larsen syndrome, a cervical spine dislocation is described and it is due to a subluxation or fusion of the vertebral bodies, usually associated with posterior vertebral arch dysraphism; the damage of the cord can cause a secondary paralysis.

5. Classification

The classification of skeletal dysplasias is based on clinical, radiographic and molecular criteria (**Figures 3** and **4**). The first international classification was established in 1969 [24]. In

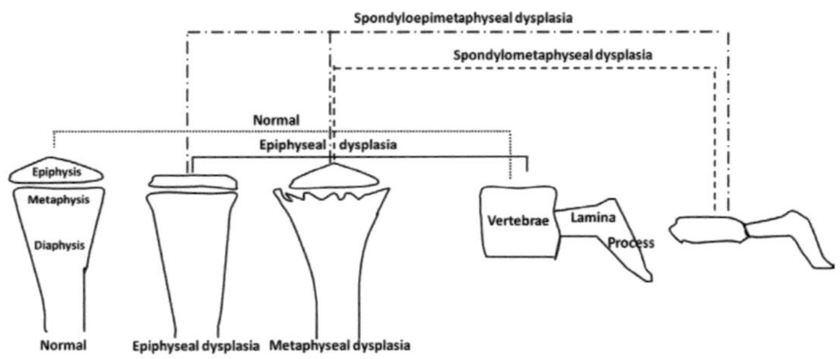

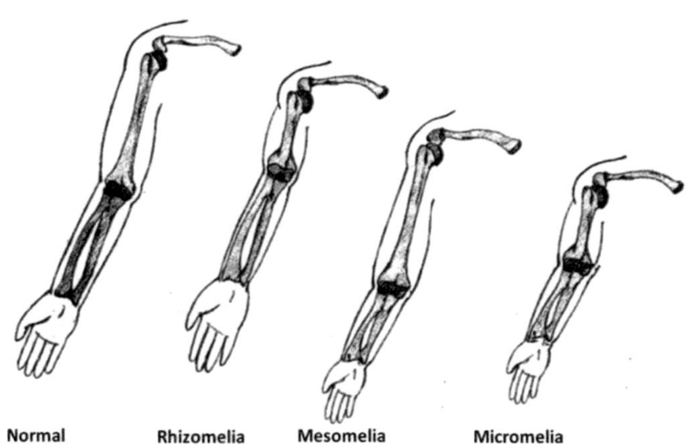

Figures 3 and 4. Cartoons that show the different portions of the appendicular skeleton that manifest radiographic abnormalities aiding in the clinical classification of the skeletal dysplasias.

http://dx.doi.org/10.5772/64802

1992, the diseases were grouped depending on radiological similarities [25], based on the concept of families proposed by Spranger (1985). Since then, the integration of clinical and radiological aspect of skeletal dysplasia was helpful in identification of disease-related genes. Gradually, phenotypically overlapping diseases were separated in different families depending on the rearranged genes. As substantial advances have been made in molecular and genetic field, classification and nomenclature must be constantly updated. The most recent classification has been made by Bonafe et al. in Nosology and Classification of Genetic Skeletal Disorders: 2015 Revision [3].

Based on the epidemiological and clinical aspects, skeletal dysplasias can be further subdivided in order to simplify the diagnostic approach [26, 27]:

- Depending on the neonatal lethality:
  - Usually fatal
    - Achondrogenesis
    - Thanatophoric dysplasia
    - Short rib polydactyly
    - Homozygous achondroplasia
    - Camptomelic dysplasia
    - Dyssegmental dysplasia, Silverman-Handmaker type
    - Osteogenesis imperfecta, type II
    - Hypophosphatasia (congenital form)
    - Chondrodysplasia punctate (rhizomelic form)
  - Often fatal
    - Asphyxiating thoracic dystrophy (jeune syndrome)
  - Occasionally fatal
    - Ellis-van Creveld syndrome
    - Diastrophic dysplasia
    - Metatropic dwarfism
    - Kniest dysplasia
- Recognizable at birth or within first month of life:
  - Most common
    - Achondroplasia
    - Osteogenesis imperfecta (types I, III, IV)

        - Spondyloepiphyseal dysplasia congenital
        - Diastrophic dysplasia
        - Ellis-van Creveld syndrome
    - Less common
        - Chondrodysplasia punctate
        - Kniest dysplasia
        - Metatropic dysplasia
        - Langer mesomelic dysplasia

5.1. Radiological features

To evaluate dysplastic patients, plain films of the entire skeleton should be evaluated (**Figures 5–10**).

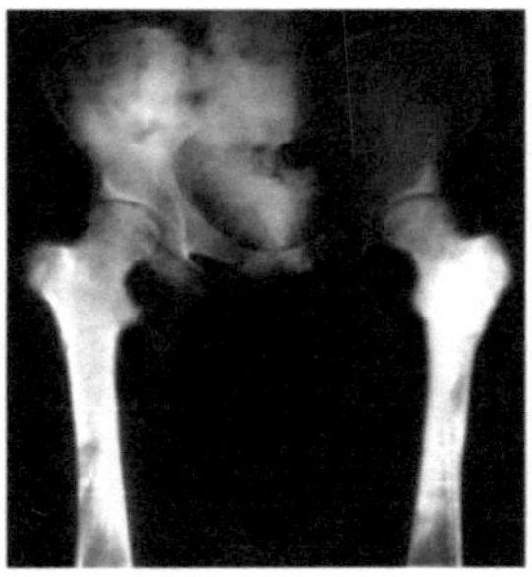

Figure 5. Achondroplasia. Squared and short ilia.

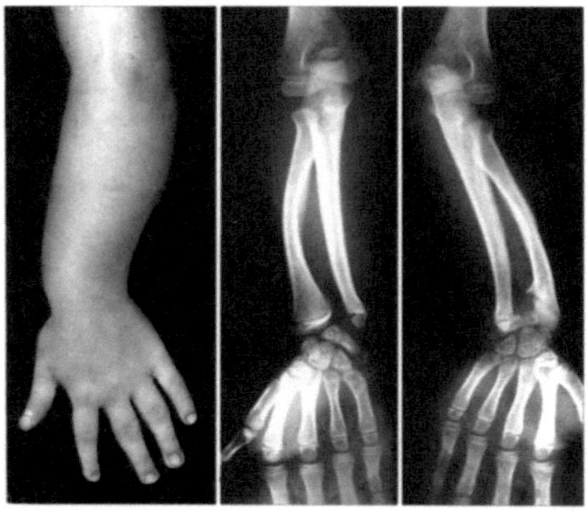

Figure 6. Leri-Weill dyschondrosteosis. Short forearms and bowing radius.

http://dx.doi.org/10.5772/64802

- As suggested by Amaka et al., a systematic approach to the skeletal survey has to be maintained. At first, it is important to define the anatomical localization of the abnormalities. Particularly, alteration of appendicular skeleton can involve the epiphysis, metaphysis or diaphysis; depending on the part involved, shortening of appendix is called rhizomelic, if proximal, mesomelic, if in the middle, acromelic, if distal or micromelic, if there is a generalized shortening of the limb. Finding very small epiphysis (due to a delay in ossification) or irregularly ossified epiphysis, radiologically suggest an epiphyseal dysplasia. Instead, the widening, the cortical thickening or the expansion/reduction of marrow space are characteristics of a diaphyseal dysplasia. The diagnosis of metaphyseal dysplasia is done if a widened, flared or irregular methapysis is found [28]. If even the spine is involved, these pathologies can be further differentiated in spondyloepiphyseal, spondylometaphyseal dysplasias [SMDs], or spondyloepimetaphyseal dysplasias [SEMDs] [2].

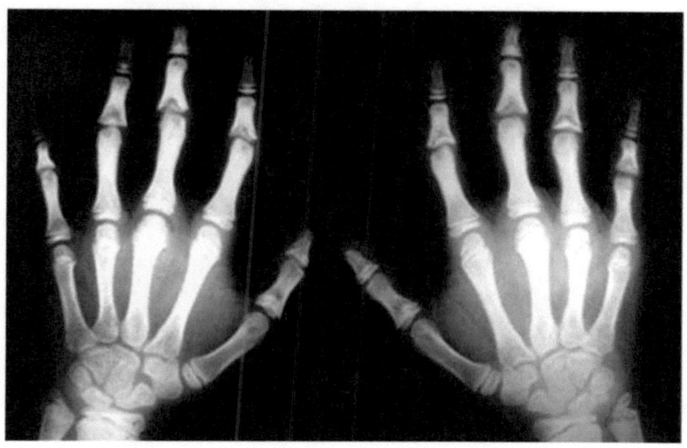

Figure 7. Trichorhinophalangeal syndrome I. Short metacarpals, especially the fourth and fifth; cone-shaped epiphyses.

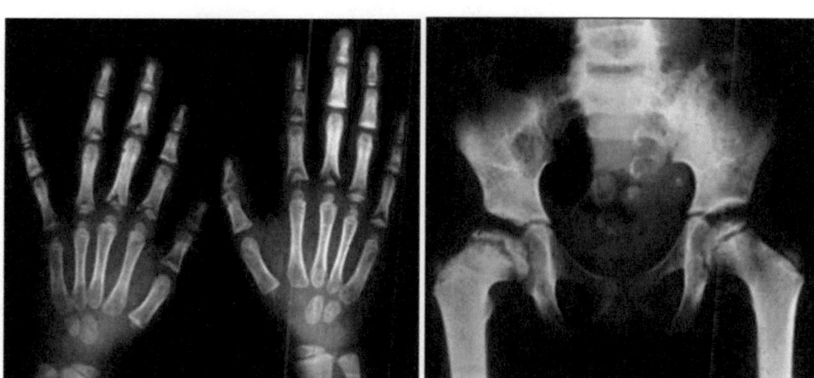

Figure 8. Trichorhinophalangeal syndrome II. Metaphyseal hooking at the proximal ends of several of the middle phalanges. Perthes-like changes in capital femoral epiphysis.

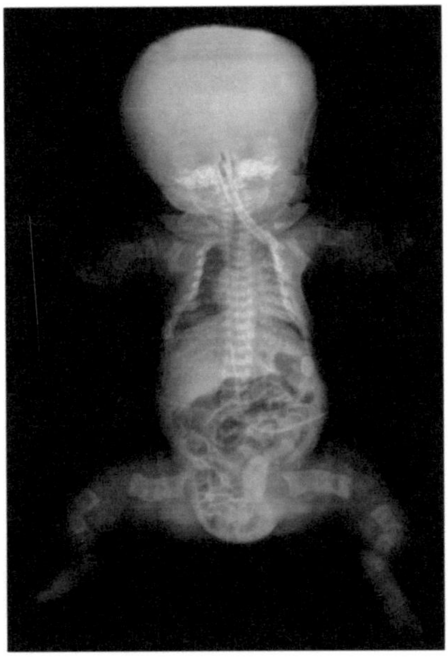

Figure 9. Type II osteogenesis imperfecta. Narrow chest. Short, broad, crumpled femora.

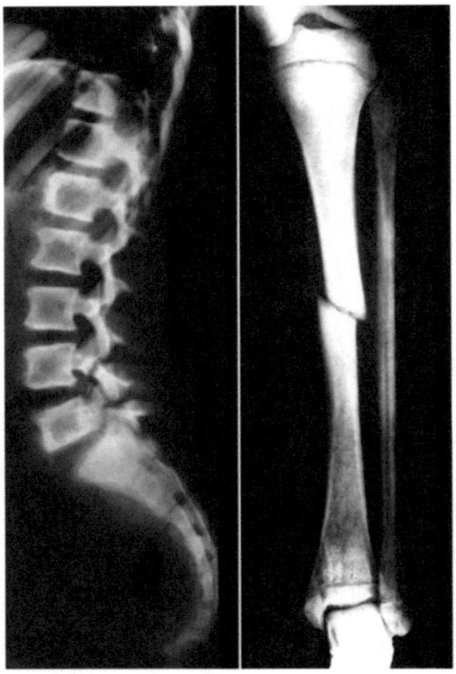

Figure 10. Pycnodysostosis. Lateral thickening of the vertebral bodies. Typical fracture of the long bone.

http://dx.doi.org/10.5772/64802

While examining the bones, the five "S" rules should be remembered:

- *Structure*: general appearance of bones, as alterations in bone density and their distribution
- *Shape*: certain bone shape is representative of specific pathologies (e.g. hooked vertebral bodies in mucopolysaccharidosis, horizontal trident acetabular roofs in achondroplasia).
- *Size*: size abnormalities can be absolute or relative to other bones. Bones can be described as tall, short, large, broad or hypoplastic
- *Sum*: the total number of bones; sometimes they are too many, too few or fuse (absent patella in nail-patella syndrome or absent radius in TAR syndrome, multiple epiphyseal centres in the patella I some form of diastrophic dysplasia)
- *Soft tissue*: wasting or excessive soft tissues, contractures and calcifications should be looked for, as they are involved in patient's prognosis.

The research of complications is important to have a complete picture of the patient. Fracture due to osteoporosis or osteopetrosis, atlantoaxial subluxation in mucopolysaccharidosis, progressive scoliosis are only few examples of the variety of the clinical scene [29].

The latest guideline about radiological classification of skeletal dysplasias points out four groups, as follow:

- GROUP 1: Epiphyseal dysplasias with/without spine involvement (Platyspondyly +/-);
- GROUP 2: Metaphyseal dysplasias with limb shortening/abnormal limb length;
- GROUP 3: Dysplasias with altered bone density;
- GROUP 4: Miscellaneous dysplasias, that is, those which do not typically have limb shortening or be clearly bracketed anatomically into sponylo-epi/metaphyseal dysplasias [28].

6. Growth in skeletal dysplasias

Skeletal dysplasias, as previously explained, affect both the linear growth and the body proportion; particularly, the growth of the legs and arms is often more compromised than the trunk [30], as well as we can discover in the ACH. In one-fourth of cases of skeletal dysplasias, the short growth is detectable since the prenatal age, while in the three-fourths remaining in the first two-three years of life. The final height is usually below 3 SD; here are presented the ranges of adult height for the most common dysplasis (**Table 2**).

Actually, the growth pattern of these rare pathologies has not been completely understood yet, because of the scarcity of data in the international literature. Therefore, it is difficult to establish whether the child grows under the standard centiles in a linearly way or if there are peculiar moment of important growth decrement. Furthermore, the same pathology can present with different phenotypes, even in the same family, thus causing other obstacle in the standardization of these children's growth.

However, because of many data regarding auxological longitudinal growth in many condition of bone dysplasia is lacking, knowledge on growth pattern is available only for a few skeletal dysplasias. It is interesting to note that different skeletal dysplasias seem to show similar growth pattern, as well as ACH, diastrophic dysplasia and cartilage-hair dysplasia. For example, in achondroplasia foetal growth is almost normal with a birth length ranging from −1.4 to 1.8 SD (**Figure 11**).

Condition	Adult height, cm
Achondroplasia	106–142 (mean: ♂ 132 cm and ♀ 125 cm)
Hypochondroplasia	132–147
Diastrophic dysplasia	86–122 (mean: ♂ 136 cm and ♀ 129 cm)
Metaphyseal dysplasia McKusick type	105–145 (mean: ♂ 131 cm and ♀ 123 cm)
Metaphyseal dysplasia Schmid type	130–160
Chondrodysplasia punctata Conradi-Hünermann type	130–160
Chondroectodermal dysplasia	106–153
Multiple epiphyseal dysplasia	137–155
Pyknodysostosis	130–150
Spondyloepiphyseal dysplasia congenital	84–132
Kniest dysplasia	104–145

Modified by [24].

Table 2. Ranges of adult height in the main skeletal dysplasia (irrespective of gender). Modified by [24].

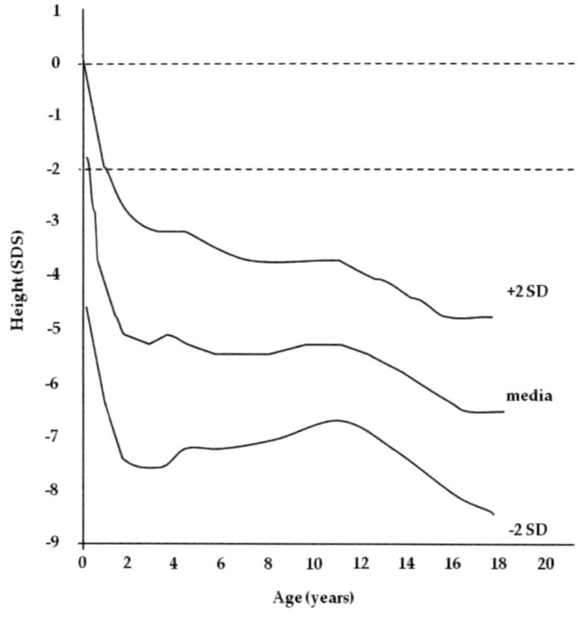

Figure 11. Mean height expressed in SDS for age in Caucasian boys and girls with achondroplasia (modified by [24]).

Hence, linear growth is fairly normal for the first postnatal months followed by a significative reduction of growth velocity and length to about –5 SD at 2 years of age. Finally, this position is maintained during the prepubertal years with a further loss during puberty (**Figure 11**).

7. Growth hormone (GH) and GH axis

The growth hormone (GH) is a polypeptide made by 191 amino acids, synthesized by somatotrope cells and stored in the anterior pituitary gland. GH is encoded by *GH1* gene situated on the long arm of chromosome 17 at position 24.2 (OMIM *139250), even if this function is regulated by a cluster of five genes strictly related. Mutations or deletions of one of these genes lead to growth hormone deficiency, resulting in short stature.

GH secretion mechanism is regulated by some hormones, principally the growth hormone releasing hormone (GHRH), the somatostatin (STT) and the Ghrelin. GHRH is a peptide produced in the hypothalamus that activates the production in and release of GH from the pituitary; GHRH binds to specific receptors, a seven transmembrane domain receptor member of the family of G-protein-coupled receptors, and located on the somatotrope cells [31]. However, STT is peptidic hormone inhibiting the release but not the GH production; STT is present in the hypothalamus but also in other part of central nervous system and in extra-nervous tissues as D-pancreatic cells, gastrointestinal cells and parafollicular thyroid cells. SST binds to a specific receptors located on the somatotrope cells, but this kind of receptors is tied to inhibitor G protein; so that way when the SST binds its receptors, it will be an inhibition of adenylate cyclase and so a decrease of c-AMP. The final result is an arrest of GH secretion from the cells.

Ghrelin, first identified in 1999 by Kojima et al. [32] is a 28 amino-acid hormone mainly synthesized in the stomach and also in the hypothalamus arcuate nucleus. Ghrelin regulation and function are very complexed, in fact it is regulated by a lot of external stimuli, such as the food intake, that decrease its secretion, instead food deprivation, hypoglycaemia and leptin administration increased this hormone [33]. Ghrelin acts directly on somatotropes cell and indirectly stimulate the release of GHRH.

GH secretion is also related to external mechanisms, such as stress, hypoglycaemia, sex hormones secretion, starvation, sleep or exercise, all condition increasing its secretion. On the contrary, other factors like hyperglycaemia, dopamine or glucocorticoid decrease it. However, many data demonstrate a bipotential action of glucocorticoid on GH secretion. In fact, while physiological level of cortisol is essential to maintain the GH axis, elevated amounts of glucocorticoid seem to increase STT levels, and so reduce GH secretion [34].

The feedback represents the most important regulatory mechanism and involves the GH, GHRH, SST and IGF-1. GH makes an auto-feedback that leads a decreased of GHRH secretion, and so that way it reduces itself. Moreover, GH stimulates SST secretion from the hypothalamus and so an ulteriore GHRH inhibition. Moreover, GHRH and SST may be able to regulate themselves reciprocally, regulating GH secretion not only acting on adenohypophysis, but also on hypothalamus. Finally, IGF-1 operates a double feedback mechanism; from one side, it inhibits GH secretion directly, and from the other side, it acts indirectly stimulating SST secretion and inhibiting GHRH secretion [34].

During the childhood GH and thyroxine are the most relevant molecules involved in linear growth; so if there is an inadequate GH secretion linear growth slows down, and we can notice a clinical short stature, usually harmonic one. However, at puberty, the activation of the hypothalamic-gonadal axis leads to a significant increase in 24-h GH, probably because of an interaction between more factors. In fact, the presence of sex hormones causes an increase of GHRH, GH and IGF-1 secretion, a decrease of SST secretion and a reduced IGF-1 negative feedback. The result is a physiological and self-limiting hypersomatotropism that it leads to the definitive stature. In this period of life, an important increase of plasma IGF-1 concentrations was observed, leading to the growth velocity peak. Then, during puberty-adult age transition, there is a decrease of GH and IGF-1 plasma concentrations [35].

8. GH-IGF-1 axis and GH treatment in skeletal dysplasias

Most patients with skeletal dysplasia show severe short stature. Surgical therapy has been attempted to correct bone deformities, but therapy conducted to improve severe short stature has been rarely attempted. However, the optimal management of physiologically and clinically heterogeneous bone disorders requires an understanding of their medical and psychosocial complications.

Syndrome	Author	Description	Outcome and results
AAA (Triple A)	Marín S. et al. (2012), [39]	A patient with a primary growth hormone (GH) insensitivity and triple A syndrome	The treatment could have had an inhibitory effect on 11β-hydroxysteroid dehydrogenase type 1 activity
Aarskog syndrome	Darendeliler F et al. (2003), [40]	The use of GH to promote growth in children with Aarskog syndrome	No adverse events were noted
Achondroplasia (ACH)	Tanaka H. (1998), [41] Liu J et al. (2015)*, [42]	GH may be beneficial in the treatment of short stature in ACH patients with subnormal GH secretion*	This may also be introduced into the medical management of ACH
Bartter syndrome	Buyukcelik M et al. (2012), [43]	Three children with Bartter syndrome and GH deficiency (GHD)	An excellent adjunctive treatment
Cartilage-hair hypoplasia (CHH)	Harada D et al. [44]	Seven years of GH treatment suggested that GH treatment significantly improved his	GH may be considered to be an efficient treatment for CHH

Syndrome	Author	Description	Outcome and results
		disturbed bone growth and had also positive efficacy to keep growth rate	
CHARGE syndrome	Esposito A et al. (2014), [45]	GHD diagnosis. GH treatment was associated with a great improvement in growth rate and resulted in a final height appropriate to his genetic target	Without any adverse event
Costello syndrome	Blachowska E et al. (2016), [46]	In cases of documented: GHD	Only under close oncologic and cardiologic supervision
Down syndrome	Annerén G et al (1999), [47]	To study the effects of GH on linear growth and psychomotor development	GH treatment ameliorates growth velocity but not affects mental or gross motor development
	Annerén G et al. (2000), [48]	15 young children with Down syndrome treated with GH	Height SDS significantly ameliorates in Down syndrome and growth velocity declined after the stop of the treatment
	Meguri K et al. (2013)*, [49]	Twenty subjects were investigated in this study*	GH is not recommended in children with Down syndrome who have not been diagnosed with GHD. GH therapy was effective for Down syndrome short stature accompanied by GHD*
Dubowitz syndrome	Hirano T et al. (1996), [50]	A child with Dubowitz syndrome, who was found to have complete GHD	He responded to GH therapy
Ellis-van Creveld syndrome (EvC)	Versteegh FG et al. (2007), [51]	Four were GHD and four were GH sufficient	In all patients treated with GH, first year growth velocity increased. In three of the four GHD and in one GH-sufficient patient a gain in height SDS was noted
Floating-Harbor syndrome (FHS)	García RJ (2012), [52]	GH treatment led to an increase in serum IGF-1 in the upper normal range,	The growth response was modest
Hypochondroplasia (HCH)	Tanaka N et al. (2003), [53]	Comparison with ACH	Short-term GH treatment in HCH is effective to increase growth rate
IMAGe	Pedreira CC et al. (2004), [54]	A patient with isolated GHD	
Kearns-Sayre syndrome	Berio A et al. (2013) [55]	A case with partial GHD	

Syndrome	Author	Description	Outcome and results
Mandibuloacral dysplasia	Agarwal AK et al. (2008), [56]	GH therapy from the ages of 3–7 years	Did not improve the short stature
Meier-Gorlin syndrome	de Munnik SA et al. (2012), [57]		GH therapy (n = 9) was generally ineffective, though in two patients with significantly reduced IGF1 levels, growth was substantially improved by GH treatment, with 2SD and 3.8 SD improvement in height
Monosomy 18p	Schober E et al.(1995), [58]		Excellent response to GH-treatment
Netherton	Aydın BK (2014), [59]	Three patients with NS who had growth retardation associated with GHD	Responded well to GH therapy
Osteogenesis imperfecta	Antoniazzi et al. [60]	30 prepubertal children with OI (type I, IV, and III) being treated with neridronate and GH	The combined rGH-Bp treatment may give better results than Bp treatment alone, in terms of BMD, lumbar spine projected area and growth velocity, particularly in patients with quantitative defects
PHACE	Merheb M et al. (2010), [61]	Improved her growth rate	Good clinical outcome
Prader-Willi syndrome	Bakker NEJ (2015), [62] Deal CL et al. (2013)*, [63]	A randomized controlled trial and longitudinal study A systematic review*	Beneficial effect of GH treatment on health-related quality of life in children with Prader-Willi syndrome Exclusion criteria should include severe obesity, uncontrolled diabetes mellitus, untreated severe obstructive sleep apnea, active cancer, or psychosis*
Pycnodysostosis	Karamizadeh Z et al. (2014), [64]	8 children. All of the patients had GHD	Positive impact on the linear growth
RASopathies	Tamburrino F et al. (2015), [65]	Starting early during childhood, resulted in a positive height response compared with untreated patients	No significant change in bone age velocity, body proportions, or cardiovascular function was observed
Ring chromosome 15	Nuutinen M wt al. (1995), [66]	severe growth retardation is a major finding	The good growth response

http://dx.doi.org/10.5772/64802

Syndrome	Author	Description	Outcome and results
Ring chromosome 18	Thomas JV et al. (2006), [67]	GHD was made due to low GH levels	The hGH therapy did not improve growth velocity
SHOX deficiency Leri-Weill dyschondrosteosis, and Langer mesomelic dysplasia	Blum WF, (2013), [68] Lughetti L et al. (2010), [69]		Similar long-term efficacy as seen in girls with TS
Silver-Russell syndrome	Binder G (2013), [70]		GH improved adult height in SRS to a comparable degree
Smith-Magenis syndrome	Itoh M et al. (2004), [71] Spadoni E et al. (2004)*, [72]	GHD could be involved in sleep disturbance in SMS. GH deficiency*	After starting replacement therapy, growth has significantly improved
Three-M syndrome	Meazza C (2013), [73]	Early start of therapy	Good compliance
Trichorhinophalangeal syndrome	Marques JS et al. (2015), [74] Riedl S et al. (2004), [75]	If the growth velocity below the normal range expected for their age and sex	Increase of growth velocity*
Turner syndrome	Tai S et al. (2013), [76] Ranke MB (2015), [77]	GH treatment in Japanese children with GHD or TS resulted in increased growth over a 4-year treatment period with a favourable safety profile.	The improvements in growth declined with time
Wolf-Hirschhorn syndrome	Titomanlio L et al. (2004), [78]	A partial GHD	GH therapy should be further considered in WHS patients

Table 3. Effects of r-hGH in some genetic syndromes and disorders.

While researchers make progress in understanding the molecular mechanisms behind these disorders and identify possible therapeutic interventions in patients with skeletal dysplasia, it remains to be identified which treatments may allow a better improvement in stature. For example, for those with achondroplasia and related disorders, fibroblast growth factor receptor 3 (FGFR3) has been identified as a critical regulator of endochondral bone growth, and in these patients mutations in the coding sequence of the *FGFR3* gene have been identified [36, 37]. In these patients, several approaches to reduce FGFR3 signalling by blocking receptor activation or inhibiting downstream signals have been proposed, some promising in preclinical animal models and other in humans [38]. In this regard, more data are available on the GH-IGF-1 axis in patients with skeletal dysplasias and genetic syndrome and GH treatment (**Table 3**). So, in this section of the chapter, we try to critically evaluate the data available on the endocrine characteristics and response to GH treatment of these patients, considering the great diversity of the studies performed as well as length of observation, the sample size and GH dosage used (**Table 3**).

8.1. Achondroplasia

ACH is characterized by short-limbed dwarfism, macrocephaly with a prominent forehead and midface hypoplasia. In ACH adult, height may be 118–145 cm for men and 112–136 cm for women [79], causing considerable inconvenience in daily life and places considerable psychological problems on patients and their families [41]. In these patients, pathogenesis involves a defective endochondral ossification while periosteal and membranous ossification are normal [80].

Many data are available about the endocrine features of ACH patients. For example, Yamate et al. [81], studying 22 patients with ACH (7 males and 15 females: age range 3–12 years), reported that at study entry, the *z*-score of their height was −5.4 ± 1.2 SD, and that of their annual height gain before admission was −3.1 ± 1.3 SD. In these patients, GH response to provocative tests was normal in more than 75%: in the patients with blunted GH secretion, 80% showed subnormal response to L-Dopa stimuli, and 20% to GHRH stimuli. A 14% of patients showed a low mean GH concentration during sleep, presenting also a markedly low IGF-1 level and marked delay of bone age [81]. However, these data were confirmed by a very large study involving 42 patients with ACH, in which it was shown that some patients presented a blunted response on different GH provocation tests, whereas other patients showed a combination of a blunted response on one provocation test and low GH concentration during sleep [41]. These authors confirmed also that some of patients showed significantly lower serum IGF-1 levels, confirming the hypothesis that a subnormal GH secretion may be discovered, even if very rarely these patients exhibited severe blunted responses (with peak GH value <5 ng/ml) to more than one type of provocation test [41].

On the contrary, data suggest that ACH children showed normal thyroid function, TSH response to TRH stimulus, as well as cortisol response to insulin-induced hypoglycaemia. In these patients, the LH and FSH responses to LHRH stimulus were also commonly appropriate to Tanner stage [41, 81].

In ACH patients, data are available about the treatment with r-hGH, even if with controversial results [41, 81–84]. Data about trials have shown a variable response to treatment, even if the limited number of patients and the variability in the pubertal stage of the enrolled subjects make it very difficult to draw any final conclusions on the role of GH therapy. Yamate et al. [81] have reported a significant increase of growth velocity compared to that before GH therapy (7.2 ± 1.4 cm/year vs. 4.1 ± 0.8 cm/year) in 18 prepubertal and pubertal ACH patients after 6 months or 1 year of GH therapy at 1 IU/kg/week. However, a 6-month therapeutical trial carried out in six patients with ACH have showed that the response may to be related on pretreatment growth velocity [84], with a greater increment of growth velocity in the patients with a lower growth rate before therapy. The authors hypothesized that the variation in response to GH therapy could be related to the different ages and pubertal stages of the enrolled children [84].

In a large study involving 42 ACH patients, Tanaka et al. showed that this significative increase of height velocity during the first year of GH treatment was reduced during the second and third years of GH therapy, although the velocity was still significant than before therapy.

http://dx.doi.org/10.5772/64802

However, the responses to GH treatment after the second year were not uniform. In these patients, the ratios of arm span to height and sitting height to overall height were not significantly increased during GH therapy, as well as there was no significant difference in mean height velocity at the end of each year between the patients with normal or subnormal GH secretion, and between the patients treated with 0.5 IU/kg per week and those treated with 1.0 IU/kg per week GH [41]. During the treatment, the authors did not show significant changes in thyroid function tests or routine laboratory data or in spinal cord compression or narrowing of the foramen magnum [41]. However, Hertel et al. [85] confirmed that, during r-hGH treatment, the mean growth velocity increased significantly during the first year reducing on the contrary below the baseline values during the third year of treatment [85]. The authors confirmed also that body proportion (sitting height/total height) or arm span did not show any significant change [85]. Besides, Weber et al. showed that short-term growth velocity increase in some but not all ACH prepubertal children, confirming the individual variability in the response to GH treatment [86]. In these patients, oral glucose tolerance test at the beginning and at the end of the therapy were in the normal range [86].

Therefore, the available data suggested that r-hGH may be useful in some patients with ACH in increasing the height and growth velocity. Waiting for new, more effective and specific treatments in patients with ACH, r-hGH treatment may be beneficial in the treatment of short stature in achondroplasia. About this, it will be helpful to the activation trials evaluating the response to different doses or also evaluate the combination of different, both medical and non-medical treatments.

8.2. Hypochondroplasia

Hypochondroplasia (HCH), a heterogeneous and usually mild form of chondrodystrophy, is a common cause of short stature. It often goes unrecognized in childhood and is diagnosed in adult life when disproportionate short stature becomes obvious [87]. Children with severe short stature and disproportion of the body segments usually have the mutation Asn540Lys [87].

The available data seem to demonstrate that patients with HCH respond to r-hGH treatment with an increase in spinal length and, coupled with a surgical leg-lengthening procedure, it is possible for some patients to achieve adult heights within the normal range [87]. However, GH therapy may restore the impairment of growth rate at puberty (**Figure 12**).

In fact, height SDS and height velocity SDS significantly improved during three-year treatment as compared with that before treatment and the improvement was much greater in HCH than in ACH [53].

Pinto et al. [88] showed that the over three-year treatment with r-hGH of 19 HCH children (11 with confirmed *FGFR3* mutations) showed an increase of height of 1.32 ± −1.05 SDS compared to untreated HCH individuals. However, Rothenbuhler et al. [89], evaluated HCH young children with confirmed *FGFR3* mutation treated with r-hGH over a six-year period. Their mean height SDS increased by 1.9 SDS, and trunk/leg disproportion was improved.

These results were confirmed by a meta-analysis involving 113 HCH children, administrated with median 0.25 mg/kg/week of r-hGH. In these patients, the therapy progressively improved the height and growth velocity with 12 months catch-up growth, and this improvement resulted constant until 36 months, even if the stature remained subnormal. While bone age chronologically progressed, no serious adverse events were reported [90].

Interestingly, using criteria based on the radiographic findings of decreased interpediculate distance between L1 and L5, Mullis et al. [91] identified two restriction fragment length polymorphisms (RFLP) within introns of IGF-1 (12q23) with a positive LOD score of 3.31 in some families with hypochondroplasia. The HCH children whose response to r-hGH treatment were characterized by a proportionate increase in both spinal and subischial leg length were all heterozygous for two co-inherited *IGF-I* gene RFLP alleles, indicating that *IGF-I* gene may be a candidate for explaining the variability in the response to r-hGH treatment [91].

In conclusion, patients with HCH seem to show a significative response to r-hGH therapy with an increase in spinal length and stature, and reduced the impaired growth spurt during puberty. It is important, therefore, to monitor all patients during childhood and give r-hGH treatment to those patients who fail to develop a growth spurt at puberty or showing a severe short stature.

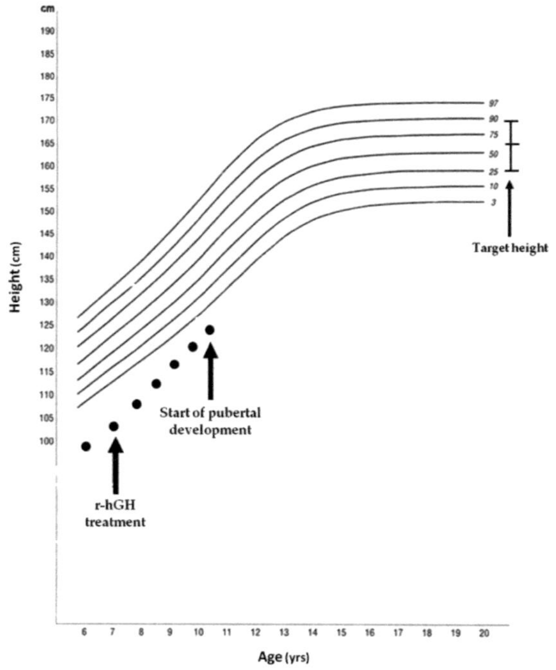

Figure 12. Effect of r-hGH therapy (the beginning is specified with the black arrow) in a female patient with a severe form of hypochondroplasia. The patients showed reduced IGF-1 and a blunted response after GH tests. You may notice the significant improvement of their stature in the short and medium term. Pubertal development onset was determined at the time of the last survey reported. X axis corresponds to the age of the patients expressed in years.

http://dx.doi.org/10.5772/64802

8.3. Type 1 trichorhinophalangeal syndrome

Type 1 trichorhinophalangeal syndrome (TRPS1), first described by Klingmuller in 1956 and then named by Giedion in 1966, is a rare genetic condition characterized by typical craniofacial and skeletal abnormalities with short stature [92]. The patients showed commonly sparse scalp hair and lateral eyebrows, bulbous tip of the nose, long flat philtrum, thin upper vermilion border and protruding ears. Skeletal abnormalities may include cone shaped epiphyses at the phalanges, hip dysplasia and short stature [92].

In TRPS1, some patients with GH deficiency have been described. Marques et al. [74] reported a 10-year-old girl with two heterozygous nonsense *TRPS1* mutations with significantly reduced growth velocity and delayed bone age. The patient shows no response to the GH stimulation tests, thus disclosed a GH deficiency, nevertheless, after r-hGH treatment catch-up growth occurred. However, Naselli et al. [93] and Sohn et al. [94] reported four unrelated patients with TRPS1 with diagnosis of GH deficiency failuring response to r-hGH treatment, whereas Stagi et al. [95] and Sarafoglou et al. [96] reported that GH treatment was effective in improving height velocity in 4 TRPS1 patients. Finally, Merjaneh et al. [97] report a TRPS1 a family with a novel nonsense mutation in the *TRPS1* gene. In this family, the eldest sibling had a normal GH-IGF-1 axis, and bone mineral density (BMD), but he accelerated his linear growth velocity over 2 years of r-hGH (0.28 mg/kg/week) increasing the height SDS score from −2.4 to −1.4. Bone age advanced by 2.5 years during 2 years of r-hGH treatment. He remained prepubertal during treatment.

The mechanism by which GH therapy could accelerate linear growth in TRPS1 is unknown. It is interesting to note that in a cell culture model mimicking *TRPS1* mutations, IGF-1

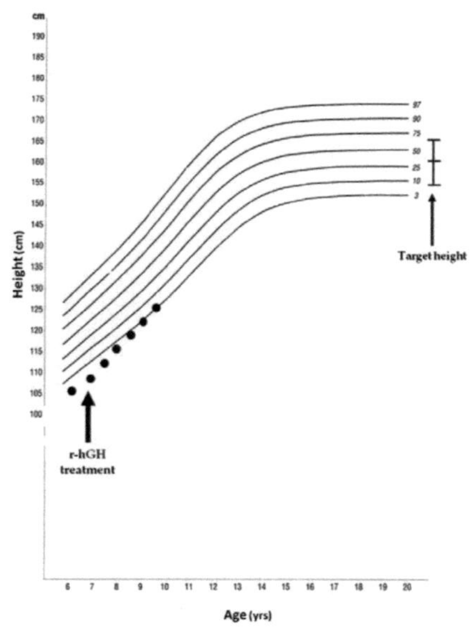

Figure 13. Effect of r-hGH therapy (the beginning is specified with the black arrow) in a female patients with type 1 Trichorhinophalangeal syndrome without GH deficiency. *X* axis corresponds to the age of the patients expressed in years.

expression was reduced by blockade of TRPS1 expression. This may suggest that the increase of IGF-1 concentrations, resulting from GH therapy, may have more effect in the growth plates of TRPS1 patients (**Figure 13**).

On the contrary, only few cases of GHD were diagnosed: a 9-year-old boy and a 10-year-old girl with TRPS2 [75, 98]. The male patient had also a TSH deficiency [99].Treatment with r-hGH was effective in both patients although their growth remained restricted. In conclusion, these data suggest performing GH stimulation tests in patients with TRPS1 or TRPS2 exhibiting a significantly reduced growth velocity and short stature. If the result is subnormal, then GH therapy should be prescribed.

8.4. Cartilage-hair hypoplasia

Cartilage-hair hypoplasia (CHH) is an autosomal recessive metaphyseal chondrodysplasia characterized by severe short-limb short stature and hypoplastic hair. The responsible gene for CHH has been identified to be *ribonuclease of mitochondrial RNA-processing* (*RMRP*) gene [99].

Bocca et al. [100] evaluated the effects of r-hGH on growth parameters and immune system in four children with CHH. The effects of treatment are more evident in patients with more severe growth retardation. However, the effects are temporary without gain in final height. However, serum immunoglobulins did not change during r-hGH treatment. On the contrary, Harada et al. [44] suggested that r-hGH treatment significantly improved the bone growth and height in CHH patients, suggesting that GH may be considered an efficient treatment for CHH. However, Obara-Moszynska et al. [101] describe another case of CHH, a girl, treated with r-hGH with a significant effect on the height gain, with an improvement from −4. to −2.98 SDS after 4 years 7 months of treatment.

In conclusion, the poor data available suggest a possible role of r-hGH in treating the severe short stature in CHH patients. However, IGF-1 and IGFBP-3 concentrations should be closely monitored during treatment, particularly because of the increased cancer risk in CHH.

8.5. Turner syndrome and short stature homeobox-containing (SHOX) gene deficiency

SHOX is the abbreviated designation for the *Short stature Homeobox-containing* gene and is localized in the pseudoautosomal region of both X and Y chromosomes [102]. *SHOX* is one of many genes that regulate longitudinal growth and SHOX deficiency, due to intragenic or regulatory region defects, cause a phenotype ranging from normal stature to mesomelic skeletal dysplasia [103].

In fact, many data showed that SHOX haploinsufficiency may be a cause of idiopathic short stature (ISS; OMIM# 604271) and the short stature of Turner syndrome (TS) patients, or Léri-Weill dyschondrosteosis (LWD; OMIM #127300), while homozygous loss of the *SHOX* gene has been related to Langer type mesomelic dysplasia (OMIM; 249700) [102].

Since discovery of *SHOX* gene in 1997, r-hGH treatment was potentially reported for growth promotion in these patients [104]. Because of SHOX deficiency represent the main cause of short stature in TS and the r-hGH acts as an efficient and safe treatment, the same therapy in short children with *SHOX* mutation at the same dosage of TS displayed an excellent growth spurt, suggesting that growth-promoting therapy with rhGH was effective with regard to height gain in short stature due to SHOX deletions [104]. In another 2-year prospective open-label randomized study involving two cohorts of SHOX-deficient patients and a cohort of TS patients, the untreated cohort grew with a normal height velocity and unchanged height SDS, whereas the r-hGH-treated cohort grew faster and as fast as the girls with TS [105]. However, retrospective data showed also that final heights in patients with SHOX deficiency treated for more than 2 years, even if with low r-hGH dose, presented an overall gain in height of 7 cm, not different from the mean gain in height in treated TS girls [106].

In conclusion, the growth-promoting effect of GH therapy, which has been approved for growth promotion in individuals with SHOX mutations by FDA and EMEA, seems to be equal to the effect reached in TS. In many patients with SHOX deficiency, an impaired GH secretion is not uncommon. r-hGH therapy is effective in increasing height in most of these patients independent of their GH secretory status, without causing any adverse events of concern.

8.6. Osteogenesis imperfecta

Osteogenesis imperfecta (OI or brittle bone disease) is a clinically and genetically heterogeneous group of heritable disorders of connective tissue [107]. The hallmark feature of OI is represented by bone fragility with susceptibility to fracture from minimal trauma. As a consequence, these patients showed bone deformity and growth deficiency [107]. However, OI patients may show other phenotypic features, as macrocephaly, blue sclerae, dentinogenesis imperfecta, hearing loss, neurological defects and cardiopulmonary complications [108].

In these patients, genetic counselling and study are essential components of complete care for individuals with OI, as are nonsurgical (e.g. rehabilitation, bracing and splinting), surgical and pharmacological (bisphosphonates or r-hGH) management [108].

In general, many data suggest that r-hGH may have a positive effect on bone growth and bone turnover by stimulating osteoblasts, collagen synthesis and longitudinal bone growth [109]; however, in the first 6 months of r-hGH therapy in GH deficiency (GHD) patients, bone resorption is usually greater than bone formation, and there are more resorption markers [110]. Besides these actions on bone GH may show a positive action on collagen metabolism [111, 112], stimulating the IGF-1 and IGFBP-3 expression, which in turn regulates the synthesis of type I collagen [113, 114].

Besides this aspect, there is scarce data about r-hGH treatment in OI patients [115–118]. Nevertheless, in one of the first attempts to treat OI patients with r-hGH, the treated patients showed, using a bone histomorphometry study, an increase in periosteal new bone formation and intracortical bone resorption, with enhanced osteoblastic activity [119]. However, the study of GH-somatomedin axis activity in OI showed that IGF-1 serum levels are frequently in the low normal range in the most part of these patients [120, 121]. In fact, Marini et al. [115]

found a hypoactivity of this axis (without a true GH deficit) in near the half of OI patients, treating them with r-hGH or clonidine. However, some data suggest that the type IV OI children would benefit from r-hGH treatment in terms of linear growth, bone matrix synthesis and bone histomorphometric parameters [122].

In a mouse model of OI, r-hGH injections [117] increased spine and femur length, produced significant changes in densitometry parameters and ameliorated the biomechanical structural properties of bone. Accordingly, similar results are obtained in human, since r-hGH treatment seems to cause a positive effect on height growth and increase in skeletal volume and BMD, with a possible subsequent reduction in fracture. However, the combined treatment with r-hGH and neridronate positively increases BMD at the lumbar spine and wrist and significantly increases the rate of linear growth velocity, with no BA advancement; and no influence in the peripheral fracture rate [60].

8.7. Ellis-van Creveld syndrome

Ellis-van Creveld syndrome (EvC; OMIM # 225500) is a skeletal dysplasia first described in 1940 by Ellis and van Creveld [123]. EvC is characterized by ectodermal dysplasia affecting mainly the teeth and nails, chondrodysplasia of the long bones, postaxial polydactyly and congenital heart anomalies. In fact, 60% of affected individuals have a congenital cardiac defect, most commonly an atrial septum defect [124]. The entity was mapped at chromosome region 4p16 [125, 126] and subsequently the *EVC* gene was cloned [127]. A second gene (*EVC2*) located in the same chromosomal region was found to harbour mutations in some EvC patients [128].

In this syndrome, data on growth patterns are limited, but in general growth is markedly impaired [51]. Growth in EvC is known to be impaired with an estimated deviation of −2.0 to −4.5 from standard growth [51]. In most reports, only one measurement of the patient is mentioned, and few follow-up data are published. In this syndrome, the GHD and the results of GH treatment were rarely reported [129].

For example, Versteegh et al. described two subjects with EvC syndrome and GHD. In the first, a mutation in the *EVC2* gene was reported. Target height was 0.28 SDS. At age 4, a decline in growth velocity was observed, and GH provocation tests disclosed a GHD. r-hGH treatment started at 2 IU/m2 resulted in improved growth velocity. Skeletal age is approximately 1 year behind at the start of r-hGH treatment, at 11 years of age exceeded the chronological age by approximately 2 years. During therapeutic GH regimens for 11 years, patient's height increased from SDS −3.3 to −1.8. In the second patients, no mutation was detected. Target height was 0.71 SDS. GHD was ruled out by an arginine stimulation test, even if, because of a severe decline in growth velocity, treatment with e-hGH was started. During 7 months of therapy, patient's height increased from −6.0 to −5.6 SDS. Versteegh et al. [51] reported also that the evaluation of the Pharmacia Growth DataBase KIGS permits to gather data on growth and GH treatment in six other EvC patients. Four patients were diagnosed as GHD. All patients except one were treated with GH according to standard protocols. A gain in height SDS was seen in three of the four GHD patients. One GHD patient did not show an increased height SDS. Of

http://dx.doi.org/10.5772/64802

the GH-sufficient, one showed a gain in height SDS. In conclusion, the available data suggest that GHD can play a role in the retarded growth in at least some EvC patients.

9. General conclusions

Skeletal dysplasias are a wild and complex group of diseases due to several pathogenetic mechanisms. Up to date, even because of their rarity, available knowledge is not so large and most of this is about a very restricted number of dysplasias. Particularly, the specific aspect of the linear growth in these patients has been analysed in a very small number of studies. No specific therapy is available and supportive measures are the only helpful treatment. By the way, data presented in literature allow us to evince that in some cases a pathological GH axis can be associated to the dysplasia. So we suggest that in this patients could be useful to investigate the function of GH axis and, if defective, to start a replacement therapy with r-hGH. Clearly, GH therapy is not a target treatment for any of these dysplasias and further studies are necessary, but it could have a supportive role in the management of the auxoendocrinological growth in these disorders.

Acknowledgements

We want to thank all the families of children with skeletal dysplasia that with love and dedication follow their children to improve their quality of life.

Competing interests: The authors declare that they have no competing interests.

Financial competing interests: The authors do not have any financial and non-financial competing interests in relation to this manuscript.

Author details

Stefano Stagi[1*], Annachiara Azzali[1], Luisa La Spina[1], Matteo Della Monica[2], Perla Scalini[1] and Maurizio de Martino[1]

*Address all correspondence to: stefano.stagi@yahoo.it

1 Department of Health Sciences, University of Florence, Anna Meyer Children's University Hospital, Florence, Italy

2 Genetics and Molecular Medicine Unit, Anna Meyer Children's University Hospital, Florence, Italy

References

[1] Cho SY, Jin DK. Guidelines for genetic skeletal dysplasias for pediatricians. Annals of Pediatric Endocrinology & Metabolism 2015;20(4):187-91.

[2] Krakow D, Rimoin DL. The skeletal dysplasias. Genetics in Medicine 2010;12(6):327-41.

[3] Bonafe L, Cormier-Daire V, Hall C, et al. Nosology and classification of genetic skeletal disorders: 2015 revision. American Journal of Medical Genetics, Part A 2015;167(12): 2869-92.

[4] Mackie EJ, Tatarczuch L, Mirams M. The skeleton: a multi-functional complex organ: the growth plate chondrocyte and endochondral ossification. The Journal of Endocrinology 2011;211(2):109-21.

[5] Mackie EJ, Ahmed YA, Tatarczuch L, et al. Endochondral ossification: how cartilage is converted into bone in the developing skeleton. The International Journal of Biochemistry & Cell Biology 2008;40(1):46-62.

[6] Yeung Tsang K, Wa Tsang S, Chan D, et al. The chondrocytic journey in endochondral bone growth and skeletal dysplasia. Birth Defects Research Part C, Embryo Today: Reviews 2014;102(1):52-73.

[7] Ricard-Blum S. The collagen family. Cold Spring Harbor Perspectives in Biology 2011;3(1):a004978.

[8] Kozhemyakina E, Lassar AB, Zelzer E. A pathway to bone: signaling molecules and transcription factors involved in chondrocyte development and maturation. Development 2015;142(5):817-31.

[9] Kronenberg HM. Developmental regulation of the growth plate. Nature 2003;423(6937):332-6.

[10] Silve C, Juppner H. Ollier disease. Orphanet Journal of Rare Diseases 2006;1:37.

[11] Emons J, Chagin AS, Savendahl L, et al. Mechanisms of growth plate maturation and epiphyseal fusion. Hormone Research in Paediatrics 2011;75(6):383-91.

[12] Nilsson O, Parker EA, Hegde A, et al. Gradients in bone morphogenetic protein-related gene expression across the growth plate. The Journal of Endocrinology 2007;193(1): 75-84.

[13] Minina E, Kreschel C, Naski MC, et al. Interaction of FGF, Ihh/Pthlh, and BMP signaling integrates chondrocyte proliferation and hypertrophic differentiation. Developmental Cell 2002;3(3):439-49.

[14] Ballock RT, Heydemann A, Wakefield LM, et al. TGF-beta 1 prevents hypertrophy of epiphyseal chondrocytes: regulation of gene expression for cartilage matrix proteins and metalloproteases. Developmental Biology 1993;158(2):414-29.

http://dx.doi.org/10.5772/64802

[15] Emons J, Chagin AS, Malmlof T, et al. Expression of vascular endothelial growth factor in the growth plate is stimulated by estradiol and increases during pubertal development. The Journal of Endocrinology 2010;205(1):61-8.

[16] Seminara S, Stagi S, Nanni L. Thyroid function during catch-up growth: a focus on the growth plate. In: The Handbook of Growth and Growth Monitoring in Health and Disease. Springer Ed., 2012. pp 905-916.

[17] Borjesson AE, Lagerquist MK, Windahl SH, et al. The role of estrogen receptor alpha in the regulation of bone and growth plate cartilage. Cellular and Molecular Life Sciences 2013;70(21):4023-37.

[18] Laurent M, Antonio L, Sinnesael M, et al. Androgens and estrogens in skeletal sexual dimorphism. Asian Journal of Andrology 2014;16(2):213-22.

[19] Vanderschueren D, Vandenput L, Boonen S, et al. Androgens and bone. Endocrine Reviews 2004;25(3):389-425.

[20] Robson H, Siebler T, Stevens DA, et al. Thyroid hormone acts directly on growth plate chondrocytes to promote hypertrophic differentiation and inhibit clonal expansion and cell proliferation. Endocrinology 2000;141(10):3887-97.

[21] Wojcicka A, Bassett JH, Williams GR. Mechanisms of action of thyroid hormones in the skeleton. Biochimica et Biophysica Acta 2013;1830(7):3979-86.

[22] von Scheven E, Corbin KJ, Stagi S, et al. Glucocorticoid-associated osteoporosis in chronic inflammatory diseases: epidemiology, mechanisms, diagnosis, and treatment. Current Osteoporosis Reports 2014;12(3):289-99.

[23] Lui JC, Baron J. Effects of glucocorticoids on the growth plate. Endocrine Development 2011;20:187-93.

[24] McKusick VA, Scott CI. A nomenclature for constitutional disorders of bone. The Journal of Bone and Joint Surgery American 1971;53(5):978-86.

[25] Beighton P, Giedion ZA, Gorlin R, et al. International classification of osteochondrodysplasias. International working group on constitutional diseases of bone. American Journal of Medical Genetics 1992;44(2):223-9.

[26] Kliegman RM. Stanton BF, St Geme JW, Schor NF. Nelson Textbook of Pediatrics. 20th ed., 2015. The skeletal dysplasias. In: Kliegman RM. Stanton BF, St Geme JW, Schor NF. Nelson Textbook of Pediatrics. 20th ed., 2015, pp 694–707.

[27] Spranger J. Pattern recognition in bone dysplasias. Progress in Clinical and Biological Research 1985;200:315-42.

[28] Panda A, Gamanagatti S, Jana M, et al. Skeletal dysplasias: a radiographic approach and review of common non-lethal skeletal dysplasias. World Journal of Radiology 2014;6(10):808-25.

[29] Offiah AC, Hall CM. Radiological diagnosis of the constitutional disorders of bone. As easy as A, B, C? Pediatric Radiology 2003;33(3):153-61.

[30] Hagenas L, Hertel T. Skeletal dysplasia, growth hormone treatment and body proportion: comparison with other syndromic and non-syndromic short children. Hormone Research 2003;60(Suppl 3):65-70.

[31] Gaylinn BD, Harrison JK, Zysk JR, et al. Molecular cloning and expression of a human anterior pituitary receptor for growth hormone-releasing hormone. Molecular Endocrinology 1993;7(1):77-84.

[32] Kojima M, Hosoda H, Date Y, et al. Ghrelin is a growth-hormone-releasing acylated peptide from stomach. Nature 1999;402(6762):656-60.

[33] Carmina E, Legro RS, Stamets K, et al. Difference in body weight between American and Italian women with polycystic ovary syndrome: influence of the diet. Human Reproduction 2003;18(11):2289-93.

[34] Giustina A, Veldhuis JD. Pathophysiology of the neuroregulation of growth hormone secretion in experimental animals and the human. Endocrine Reviews 1998;19(6): 717-97.

[35] Pincus SM, Veldhuis JD, Rogol AD. Longitudinal changes in growth hormone secretory process irregularity assessed transpubertally in healthy boys. American Journal of Physiology, Endocrinology and Metabolism 2000;279(2):E417-24.

[36] Bellus GA, Bamshad MJ, Przylepa KA, et al. Severe achondroplasia with developmental delay and acanthosis nigricans (SADDAN): phenotypic analysis of a new skeletal dysplasia caused by a Lys650Met mutation in fibroblast growth factor receptor 3. American Journal of Medical Genetics 1999;85(1): 53-65.

[37] Rousseau F, Bonaventure J, Legeai-Mallet L, et al. Mutations in the gene encoding fibroblast growth factor receptor-3 in achondroplasia. Nature 1994;371(6494):252-4.

[38] Garcia S, Dirat B, Tognacci T, et al. Postnatal soluble FGFR3 therapy rescues achondroplasia symptoms and restores bone growth in mice. Science Translational Medicine 2013;5(203):203ra124.

[39] Marín S, Casano-Sancho P, Villarreal-Peña N, et al. Triple A syndrome in a patient with genetic growth hormone insensitivity: phenotypic effects of two genetic disorders. Hormone Research in Paediatrics 2012;77(1):63–8.

[40] Darendeliler F, Larsson P, Neyzi O, et al. Growth hormone treatment in Aarskog syndrome: analysis of the KIGS (Pharmacia International Growth Database) data. Journal of Pediatric Endocrinology & Metabolism 2003;16(8):1137–42.

http://dx.doi.org/10.5772/64802

[41] Tanaka H, Kubo T, Yamate T, et al. Effect of growth hormone therapy in children with achondroplasia: Growth pattern, hypothalamic-pituitary function, and genotype. European Journal of Endocrinology 1998;138(3):275–80.

[42] Liu J, Tang X, Cheng J, Wang L, et al. Analysis of the clinical and molecular characteristics of a child with achondroplasia: a case report. Experimental and Therapeutic Medicine 2015;9(5):1763–7.

[43] Buyukcelik M, Keskin M, Kilic BD, et al. Bartter syndrome and growth hormone deficiency: three cases. Pediatric Nephrology 2012;27(11):2145–8.

[44] Harada D, Yamanaka Y, Ueda K, et al. An effective case of growth hormone treatment on cartilage-hair hypoplasia. Bone 2005;36(2):317–22.

[45] Esposito A, Tufano M, Di Donato I, et al. Effect of long-term GH treatment in a patient with CHARGE association. Italian Journal of Pediatrics 2014;40:51.

[46] Blachowska E, Petriczko E, Horodnicka-Józwa A, et al. Recombinant growth hormone therapy in a girl with Costello syndrome: a 4-year observation. Italian Journal of Pediatrics 2016;42(1):10.

[47] Annerén G, Tuvemo T, Carlsson-Skwirut C, et al. Growth hormone treatment in young children with Down's syndrome: effects on growth and psychomotor development. Archives of Disease in Childhood 1999;80(4):334–8.

[48] Annerén G, Tuvemo T, Gustafsson J. Growth hormone therapy in young children with Down syndrome and a clinical comparison of Down and Prader-Willi syndromes. Growth Hormone & IGF Research 2000;10 Suppl B:S87–91.

[49] Meguri K, Inoue M, Narahara K, et al. Therapeutic efficacy and safety of GH in Japanese children with Down syndrome short stature accompanied by GH deficiency. Clinical Pediatric Endocrinology 2013;22(4):65–72.

[50] Hirano T, Izumi I, Tamura K. Growth hormone deficiency in Dubowitz syndrome. Acta Paediatrica Japonica 1996;38(3):267–9.

[51] Versteegh FG, Buma SA, Costin G, et al. Growth hormone analysis and treatment in Ellis-van Creveld syndrome. American Journal of Medical Genetics Part A 2007;143A(18):2113-21.

[52] García RJ, Kant SG, Wit JM, et al. Clinical and genetic characteristics and effects of long-term growth hormone therapy in a girl with Floating-Harbor syndrome. Journal of Pediatric Endocrinology & Metabolism 2012;25(1-2):207–12.

[53] Tanaka N, Katsumata N, Horikawa R, et al. The comparison of the effects of short-term growth hormone treatment in patients with achondroplasia and with hypochondroplasia. Endocrine Journal 2003;50(1):69–75.

[54] Pedreira CC, Savarirayan R, Zacharin MR. IMAGe syndrome: a complex disorder affecting growth, adrenal and gonadal function, and skeletal development. The Journal of Pediatrics 2004;144(2):274–7.

[55] Berio A, Piazzi A. Multiple endocrinopathies (growth hormone deficiency, autoimmune hypothyroidism and diabetes mellitus) in Kearns-Sayre syndrome. La Pediatria Medica e Chirurgica. 2013;35(3):137–40.

[56] Agarwal AK, Kazachkova I, Ten S, et al. Severe mandibuloacral dysplasia-associated lipodystrophy and progeria in a young girl with a novel homozygous Arg527Cys LMNA mutation. The Journal of Clinical Endocrinology and Metabolism 2008;93(12): 4617–23.

[57] de Munnik SA, Otten BJ, Schoots J, et al. Meier-Gorlin syndrome: growth and secondary sexual development of a microcephalic primordial dwarfism disorder. American Journal of Medical Genetics. Part A 2012;158A(11):2733–42.

[58] Schober E, Scheibenreiter S, Frisch H. 18p monosomy with GH-deficiency and empty sella: good response to GH-treatment. Clinical Genetics 1995;47(5):254–6.

[59] Aydın BK, Baş F, Tamay Z, et al. Netherton syndrome associated with growth hormone deficiency. Pediatric Dermatology 2014;31(1):90–4.

[60] Antoniazzi F, Monti E, Venturi G, et al. GH in combination with bisphosphonate treatment in osteogenesis imperfecta. European Journal of Endocrinology 2010;163(3): 479–87.

[61] Merheb M, Hourani R, Zantout MS, et al. Endocrine dysfunction in a patient with PHACE syndrome, including port-wine stain of the right periorbital area. Endocrine Practice 2010;16(2):255–9.

[62] Bakker NE, Siemensma EP, van Rijn M, et al. Beneficial effect of growth hormone treatment on health-related quality of life in children with Prader-Willi syndrome: A Randomized Controlled Trial and Longitudinal Study. Hormone Research in Paediatrics 2015;84(4):231–9.

[63] Deal CL, Tony M, Höybye C, et al. Growth Hormone Research Society workshop summary: consensus guidelines for recombinant human growth hormone therapy in Prader-Willi syndrome. The Journal of Clinical Endocrinology and Metabolism 2013;98(6):E1072–87.

[64] Karamizadeh Z, Ilkhanipoor H, Bagheri F. Effect of growth hormone treatment on height velocity of children with pycnodysostosis. Iranian Journal of Pediatrics 2014;24(2):161–5.

[65] Tamburrino F, Gibertoni D, Rossi C, et al. Response to long-term growth hormone therapy in patients affected by RASopathies and growth hormone deficiency: patterns of growth, puberty and final height data. American Journal of Medical Genetics. Part A 2015;167A(11):2786–94.

[66] Nuutinen M, Kouvalainen K, Knip M. Good growth response to growth hormone treatment in the ring chromosome 15 syndrome. Journal of Medical Genetics 1995;32(6): 486–7.

[67] Thomas JV, Mezzasalma DF, Teixeira AM, et al. [Growth hormone deficiency, hypothyroidism and ring chromosome 18: case report]. Arquivos Brasileiros de Endocrinologia e Metabologia. 2006;50(5):951–6.

[68] Blum WF, Ross JL, Zimmermann AG, et al., GH treatment to final height produces similar height gains in patients with SHOX deficiency and Turner syndrome: results of a multicenter trial. The Journal of Clinical Endocrinology and Metabolism 2013;98(8):E1383–92.

[69] Iughetti L, Madeo S, Predieri B. Growth hormone therapy in patients with short stature homeobox-gene (SHOX) deficiency. Journal of Endocrinological Investigation 2010;33(6 Suppl):34–8.

[70] Binder G, Liebl M, Woelfle J, et al. Adult height and epigenotype in children with Silver-Russell syndrome treated with GH. Hormone Research in Paediatrics 2013;80(3):193–200.

[71] Itoh M, Hayashi M, Hasegawa T, et al. Systemic growth hormone corrects sleep disturbance in Smith-Magenis syndrome. Brain and Development 2004;26(7):484–6.

[72] Spadoni E, Colapietro P, Bozzola M, et al. Smith-Magenis syndrome and growth hormone deficiency. European Journal of Pediatrics 2004;163(7):353–8.

[73] Meazza C, Lausch E, Pagani S, et al., 3-M syndrome associated with growth hormone deficiency: 18 year follow-up of a patient. Italian Journal of Pediatrics 2013;39:21.

[74] Marques JS, Maia C, Almeida R, et al. Should patients with Trichorhinophalangeal syndrome be tested for growth hormone deficiency? Pediatric Endocrinology Reviews: 2015;13(1):465–7.

[75] Riedl S, Giedion A, Schweitzer K, et al. Pronounced short stature in a girl with tricho-rhino-phalangeal syndrome II (TRPS II, Langer-Giedion syndrome) and growth hormone deficiency. American Journal of Medical Genetics Part A 2004;131(2):200–3.

[76] Tai S, Tanaka T, Hasegawa T, et al. An observational study of the effectiveness and safety of growth hormone (Humatrope(®)) treatment in Japanese children with growth hormone deficiency or Turner syndrome. Endocrine Journal 2013;60(1):57–64.

[77] Ranke MB. Why treat girls with Turner syndrome with growth hormone? Growth and beyond. Pediatric Endocrinology Reviews 2015;12(4):356–65.

[78] Titomanlio L, Romano A, Conti A, et al. Mild Wolf-Hirschhorn phenotype and partial GH deficiency in a patient with a 4p terminal deletion. American Journal of Medical Genetics: Part A 2004;127A(2):197–200.

[79] Horton WA, Rotter JI, Rimoin DL, et al. Standard growth curves for achondroplasia. The Journal of Pediatrics 1978;93(3):435-8.

[80] Rimoin DL, Hughes GN, Kaufman RL, et al. Endochondral ossification in achondroplastic dwarfism. The New England Journal of Medicine 1970;283(14):728-35.

[81] Yamate T, Kanzaki S, Tanaka H, et al. Growth hormone (GH) treatment in achondroplasia. The Journal of Pediatric Endocrinology 1993;6(1):45-52.

[82] Nishi Y, Kajiyama M, Miyagawa S, et al. Growth hormone therapy in achondroplasia. Acta Endocrinologica 1993;128(5):394-6.

[83] Okabe T, Nishikawa K, Miyamori C, et al. Growth-promoting effect of human growth hormone on patients with achondroplasia. Acta Paediatrica Japonica 1991;33(3):357-62.

[84] Horton WA, Hecht JT, Hood OJ, et al. Growth hormone therapy in achondroplasia. American Journal of Medical Genetics 1992;42(5):667-70.

[85] Hertel NT, Eklof O, Ivarsson S, et al. Growth hormone treatment in 35 prepubertal children with achondroplasia: a five-year dose-response trial. Acta Paediatrica 2005;94(10):1402-10.

[86] Weber G, Prinster C, Meneghel M, et al. Human growth hormone treatment in prepubertal children with achondroplasia. American Journal of Medical Genetics 1996;61(4): 396-400.

[87] Ramaswami U, Hindmarsh PC, Brook CG. Growth hormone therapy in hypochondroplasia. Acta Paediatrica 1999;88(428):116-7.

[88] Pinto G, Cormier-Daire V, Le Merrer M, et al. Efficacy and safety of growth hormone treatment in children with hypochondroplasia: comparison with an historical cohort. Hormone Research in Paediatrics 2014;82(6):355-63.

[89] Rothenbuhler A, Linglart A, Piquard C, et al. A pilot study of discontinuous, insulin-like growth factor 1-dosing growth hormone treatment in young children with FGFR3 N540K-mutated hypochondroplasia. The Journal of Pediatrics 2012;160(5):849-53.

[90] Massart F, Miccoli M, Baggiani A, et al. Height outcome of short children with hypochondroplasia after recombinant human growth hormone treatment: a meta-analysis. Pharmacogenomics 2015;16(17):1965-73.

[91] Mullis PE, Patel MS, Brickell PM, et al. Growth characteristics and response to growth hormone therapy in patients with hypochondroplasia: genetic linkage of the insulin-like growth factor I gene at chromosome 12q23 to the disease in a subgroup of these patients. Clinical Endocrinology 1991;34(4):265-74.

[92] Candamourty R, Venkatachalam S, Karthikeyan B, et al. Trichorhinophalangeal syndrome type 1: a case report with literature review. Journal of Natural Science, Biology, and Medicine 2012;3(2):209-11.

[93] Naselli A, Vignolo M, Di Battista E, et al. Trichorhinophalangeal syndrome type I in monozygotic twins discordant for hip pathology. Report on the morphological evolution of cone-shaped epiphyses and the unusual pattern of skeletal maturation. Pediatric Radiology 1998;28(11):851-5.

[94] Sohn YB, Ki CS, Park SW, et al. Clinical, biochemical, and genetic analysis of two Korean patients with trichorhinophalangeal syndrome type I and growth hormone deficiency. Annals of Clinical and Laboratory Science 2012;42(3):307-12.

[95] Stagi S, Bindi G, Galluzzi F, et al. Partial growth hormone deficiency and changed bone quality and mass in type I trichorhinophalangeal syndrome. American Journal of Medical Genetics Part A 2008;146A(12):1598-604.

[96] Sarafoglou K, Moassesfar S, Miller BS. Improved growth and bone mineral density in type I trichorhinophalangeal syndrome in response to growth hormone therapy. Clinical Genetics 2010;78(6):591-3.

[97] Merjaneh L, Parks JS, Muir AB, et al. A novel TRPS1 gene mutation causing trichorhinophalangeal syndrome with growth hormone responsive short stature: a case report and review of the literature. International Journal of Pediatric Endocrinology 2014;2014(1):16.

[98] Schinzel A, Riegel M, Baumer A, et al. Long-term follow-up of four patients with Langer-Giedion syndrome: clinical course and complications. American Journal of Medical Genetics Part A 2013;161A(9):2216-25.

[99] Nakhoul H, Ke J, Zhou X, et al. Ribosomopathies: mechanisms of disease. Clinical Medicine Insights Blood Disorders 2014;7:7-16.

[100] Bocca G, Weemaes CM, van der Burgt I, et al. Growth hormone treatment in cartilage-hair hypoplasia: effects on growth and the immune system. Journal of Pediatric Endocrinology & Metabolism 2004;17(1):47-54.

[101] Obara-Moszynska M, Wielanowska W, Rojek A, et al. Treatment of cartilage-hair hypoplasia with recombinant human growth hormone. Pediatrics International 2013;55(6):e162-4.

[102] Leka SK, Kitsiou-Tzeli S, Kalpini-Mavrou A, et al. Short stature and dysmorphology associated with defects in the SHOX gene. Hormones 2006;5(2):107-18.

[103] Child CJ, Kalifa G, Jones C, et al. Radiological features in patients with short stature Homeobox-Containing (SHOX) gene deficiency and Turner syndrome before and after 2 years of GH treatment. Hormone Research in Paediatrics 2015;84(1):14-25.

[104] Binder G, Schwarze CP, Ranke MB. Identification of short stature caused by SHOX defects and therapeutic effect of recombinant human growth hormone. The Journal of Clinical Endocrinology and Metabolism 2000;85(1):245-9.

[105] Blum WF, Crowe BJ, Quigley CA, et al. Growth hormone is effective in treatment of short stature associated with short stature homeobox-containing gene deficiency: Two-

year results of a randomized, controlled, multicenter trial. The Journal of Clinical Endocrinology and Metabolism 2007;92(1):219-28.

[106] Blum WF, Cao D, Hesse V, et al. Height gains in response to growth hormone treatment to final height are similar in patients with SHOX deficiency and Turner syndrome. Hormone Research 2009;71(3):167-72.

[107] Forlino A, Marini JC. Osteogenesis imperfecta. Lancet 2016;387(10028):1657–71.

[108] Marini J, Smith SM. Osteogenesis imperfecta. In: De Groot LJ, Beck-Peccoz P, Chrousos G, et al., eds. Endotext. South Dartmouth (MA), 2000.

[109] Giustina A, Mazziotti G, Canalis E. Growth hormone, insulin-like growth factors, and the skeleton. Endocrine Reviews 2008;29(5):535-59.

[110] Ohlsson C, Bengtsson BA, Isaksson OG, et al. Growth hormone and bone. Endocrine Reviews 1998;19(1):55-79.

[111] Ernst M, Rodan GA. Increased activity of insulin-like growth factor (IGF) in osteoblastic cells in the presence of growth hormone (GH): positive correlation with the presence of the GH-induced IGF-binding protein BP-3. Endocrinology 1990;127(2):807-14.

[112] McCarthy TL, Casinghino S, Centrella M, et al. Complex pattern of insulin-like growth factor binding protein expression in primary rat osteoblast enriched cultures: regulation by prostaglandin E2, growth hormone, and the insulin-like growth factors. Journal of Cellular Physiology 1994;160(1):163-75.

[113] Hock JM, Centrella M, Canalis E. Insulin-like growth factor I has independent effects on bone matrix formation and cell replication. Endocrinology 1988;122(1):254-60.

[114] Wergedal JE, Mohan S, Lundy M, et al. Skeletal growth factor and other growth factors known to be present in bone matrix stimulate proliferation and protein synthesis in human bone cells. Journal of Bone and Mineral Research 1990;5(2):179-86.

[115] Marini JC, Bordenick S, Heavner G, et al. The growth hormone and somatomedin axis in short children with osteogenesis imperfecta. The Journal of Clinical Endocrinology and Metabolism 1993;76(1):251-6.

[116] Marini JC, Hopkins E, Glorieux FH, et al. Positive linear growth and bone responses to growth hormone treatment in children with types III and IV osteogenesis imperfecta: high predictive value of the carboxyterminal propeptide of type I procollagen. Journal of Bone and Mineral Research 2003;18(2):237-43.

[117] King D, Jarjoura D, McEwen HA, et al. Growth hormone injections improve bone quality in a mouse model of osteogenesis imperfecta. Journal of Bone and Mineral Research 2005;20(6):987-93.

[118] Vieira NE, Marini JC, Hopkins E, et al. Effect of growth hormone treatment on calcium kinetics in patients with osteogenesis imperfecta type III and IV. Bone 1999;25(4):501-5.

[119] Kruse HP, Kuhlencordt F. On an attempt to treat primary and secondary osteoporosis with human growth hormone. Hormone and metabolic research = Hormon- und Stoffwechselforschung = Hormones et Metabolisme 1975;7(6):488-91.

[120] Vetter U, Pontz B, Zauner E, et al. Osteogenesis imperfecta: a clinical study of the first ten years of life. Calcified Tissue International 1992;50(1):36-41.

[121] Lund AM, Muller J, Skovby F. Anthropometry of patients with osteogenesis imperfecta. Archives of Disease in Childhood 1999;80(6):524-8.

[122] Letocha AD, Cintas HL, Troendle JF, et al. Controlled trial of pamidronate in children with types III and IV osteogenesis imperfecta confirms vertebral gains but not short-term functional improvement. Journal of Bone and Mineral Research 2005;20(6):977-86.

[123] Shetty P, Shetty D, Priyadarshana PS, et al. A rare case report of Ellis Van Creveld syndrome in an Indian patient and literature review. Journal of Oral Biology and Craniofacial Research 2015;5(2):98-101.

[124] Verbeek S, Eilers PH, Lawrence K, et al. Growth charts for children with Ellis-van Creveld syndrome. European Journal of Pediatrics 2011;170(2):207-11.

[125] Polymeropoulos MH, Ide SE, Wright M, et al. The gene for the Ellis-van Creveld syndrome is located on chromosome 4p16. Genomics 1996;35(1):1-5.

[126] Howard TD, Guttmacher AE, McKinnon W, et al. Autosomal dominant postaxial polydactyly, nail dystrophy, and dental abnormalities map to chromosome 4p16, in the region containing the Ellis-van Creveld syndrome locus. American Journal of Human Genetics 1997;61(6):1405-12.

[127] Ruiz-Perez VL, Ide SE, Strom TM, et al. Mutations in a new gene in Ellis-van Creveld syndrome and Weyers acrodental dysostosis. Nature Genetics 2000;24(3):283-6.

[128] Galdzicka M, Patnala S, Hirshman MG, et al. A new gene, EVC2, is mutated in Ellis-van Creveld syndrome. Molecular Genetics and Metabolism 2002;77(4):291-5.

[129] Cacciari E, Pirazzoli P, Mandini M. GH therapy in two patients with osteochondrodysplasia. Basic Life Sciences 1988;48:129-33.

Section 2

Genetics and Diagnosis of Restricted Growth

Chapter 2

Growth Hormone Deficiency: Diagnosis and Therapy in Children

Mauro Bozzola and Cristina Meazza

Additional information is available at the end of the chapter

http://dx.doi.org/10.5772/64803

Abstract

Short stature has been defined as a height below the 2 standard deviation for age, sex and ethnicity. Growth hormone deficiency (GHD) represents a condition characterized by reduced GH secretion, isolated or associated with other pituitary hormone deficiencies. In a child with short stature and growth deceleration, after the exclusion of other causes of growth failure, the diagnosis of GHD has to be confirmed by measurement of GH secretion after at least two stimulation tests. Patients with GHD should be treated with rhGH as soon as possible, to obtain normalization of growth and normal final height. The catch-up growth in response to rhGH therapy is maximal during the first years and could be affected by many variables, such as birth-weight, age and height at start of treatment and of puberty, and duration of treatment. Overall rhGH is believed to be safe and significant side-effects in children are very rare, including benign intracranial hypertension, hyperglycaemia, arthralgia and myalgia. Patients with childhood onset GHD are usually retested in late adolescence to confirm the GHD persistence and to continue of GH therapy. In conclusion, the present chapter provides useful and updated information about the diagnosis, treatment and follow-up of children with GHD.

Keywords: growth hormone, growth hormone deficiency, GH substitutive therapy, children, multiple pituitary hormone deficiency

1. Introduction

Human height is regulated by interactions among different factors such as genetic predisposition, nutritional status, hormonal secretion and environmental factors. Traditionally, short stature has been defined as a height of two standard deviations (SD) below the mean of sex, age and ethnic-matched healthy controls, and is a frequent reason for referral to paediatric endocrinologists [1, 2]. Growth hormone deficiency (GHD) is a rare but important cause of short stature with a prevalence of approximately of one in 4000 during childhood [3]. Although it is a rare condition, it is important to make a correct diagnosis in order to promptly start substitutive recombinant human (rh) GH therapy and obtain a normalization of child growth. In fact, missing a diagnosis will result in poor growth and short stature adults. On the other hand, a false positive diagnosis will lead to many years of daily subcutaneous injections and significant unnecessary expenditure.

2. Growth hormone deficiency

Growth hormone deficiency is classically defined as insufficient GH secretion that results in a decrease in the production of GH-dependent hormones and growth factors, such as insulin-like growth factor-I (IGF-I), IGF-II and their binding proteins (IGFBPs) [4].

Growth hormone deficiency may be isolated or combined with other pituitary hormone deficiencies (CPHD, combined pituitary hormone deficiency) and may be congenital or acquired [5]. Acquired GHD may be secondary to hypothalamic-pituitary damage at birth or intracranial neoplasm (i.e. craniopharyngioma), infiltrative diseases (i.e. Langerhans cell histiocytosis), infections (i.e. tuberculosis, HIV), trauma, cranial or total body irradiation (TBI) and chemotherapy.

In most cases, GHD is idiopathic and only in 20% of patients an organic cause is identified. Among idiopathic cases, abnormalities in magnetic resonance imaging (MRI) of hypothalamic-pituitary region are frequent (pituitary hypoplesia, lack of pituitary stalk, ectopic posterior pituitary) [6, 7]. In some cases of GHD, an autoimmune origin may be hypothesized based on the detection of circulating anti-pituitary antibodies directed against GH-secreting cells. Anti-pituitary antibodies have also been detected in some patients with idiopathic short stature, who subsequently showed impaired GH secretion suggestive of a particular type of acquired GHD [8].

2.1. Genetics defect in isolated GHD

Gene defects have been associated with GHD (**Table 1**). Mutations have been found in the genes encoding for GH (*GH1*) or GH releasing hormone receptor (*GHRHR*). *GH1* mutations can either lead to classic GHD (types IA, IB and II) or bio-inactive GH syndrome, a condition characterized by normal or elevated circulating not active GH levels [9]. Homozygous *GH1* deletions are a common cause of type IA GHD and patients can develop anti-GH antibodies during GH therapy. Type IB GHD is a less severe form and is caused by mutations of *GH1* or *GHRHR*, while GHD type II is a dominant form caused by skipping of exon 3 which results in the secretion of a GH isoform (17.5 kDa) with a dominant negative effect [10]. Furthermore, the X-linked type III GHD is associated with agammaglobulinemia and has been associated with mutations in *BTK* and *SOX3* genes [11, 12]. Another cause of GHD could be mutations of the gene encoding for the ghrelin receptor (GHSR), which decrease in GH secretion [13].

Disorder*	Gene(s)	Inheritance	Clinical features/GH levels	Response to GH therapy	References
Isolated GHD type IB (612781)	GHRHR	AR	Low serum GH	Positive	[106, 107]
Isolated GHD type IA (262400)	GH1	AR	No serum GH	Often anti-GH antibodies	[106, 107]
Isolated GHD type IB (612781)	GH1	AR	Low serum GH	Positive	[106, 107]
Isolated GHD type II (173100)	GH1	AD	Variable height deficit and pituitary size; low GH levels; other pituitary deficits can develop	Positive	[106, 107]
Isolated GHD type III (307200)	BTK, SOX3	XLR	Low GH levels with agammaglobulinaemia	Positive	[106, 107]
Isolated partial GHD(615925)	GHSR	AR, AD	Variable serum GH and IGF-I	No data	[13, 108]
Almstrom syndrome (203800)	ALMS1	AR	50% of cases are GHD	No data	[16]
	RNPC3	AR	Severe GHD, hypoplasia anterior pituitary	No data	[14]
	IFT172	AR	Functional GHD, retinopathy, metaphyseal dysplasia, hypertension	Positive	[15]

*Name (number) according to OMIM.

Abbreviations: AD, autosomal dominant; AR, autosomal recessive; XLR, X-linked recessive.

Table 1. Gene defects associated with isolated GHD.

Finally, many studies reported isolated GHD associated with congenital syndromes caused by mutations and/or deletions of different genes not directly involved in growth (i.e. biallelic mutations in *RNPC3*, compound heterozygosity for *IFT172* or mutation of *ALMS1*) [14–16].

2.2. Genetics of combined pituitary hormone deficiency

In childhood, some patients may show GHD associated with deficiency of other pituitary hormones such as prolactin, thyroid stimulating hormone (TSH), luteinizing hormone (LH) and follicle-stimulating hormone (FSH), and, sometimes, adrenocorticotropic hormone (ACTH) [4].

Several genetic defects of transcription factors have been reported in CPHD (**Table 2**). Two categories of patients with hypopituitarism are described according to the presence or absence of extra-pituitary abnormalities and/or malformations, beside anterior pituitary hormone deficiencies [17]. The phenotypes with heterogeneous extra-pituitary abnormalities are caused by mutations in transcription factor genes early expressed in regions determining the formation of forebrain and related midline structures, such as hypothalamus and pituitary. Defects have been found in *SHH, FGFR1* and *FGF8, LHX3* and *LHX4, HESX1, SOX2* and *SOX3, OTX2, PROK2* and *PROKR2, PITX2* and many others [18]. On the other hand, phenotypes without any extra-pituitary malformations are due to mutations of late-acting pituitary-specific transcription factors. Mutations in transcription factors such as *POU1F-1* and *PROP-1* are commonly linked to deficiency of GH, TSH, LH, FSH and sometimes ACTH [19]. Furthermore, as recently described by Giordano et al., deletions of particular chromosome regions including these genes lead to syndromes often associated with isolated GHD or CPHD [20].

Disorder*	Gene(s)	Clinical features	Inheritance	References
CPHD-1 (613038)	POU1F1	GH, PRL, variable TSH deficiency	AR, AD	[18, 109, 110]
CPHD-2 (262600)	PROP1	GH, PRL, TSH, LH, FSH, variable ACTH deficiency	AR	[18, 109, 110]
CPHD-3 (221750)	LHX3	GH, PRL, TSH, LH, FSH deficiency	AR	[18, 109, 110]
CPHD-4 (262700)	LHX4	GH, TSH, ACTH deficiency	AD, AR	[18, 109, 110]
Septo-optic dysplasia (CPHD-5) (182230)	HESX1	Optic nerve and pituitary hypoplasia, midline abnormalities of brain, TSH, GH, PRL, LH, FSH and ACTH deficiency	AR, AD	[18, 109, 110]
CPHD-6 (613986)	OTX2	GH, TSH, LH, FSH, variable ACTH and PRL	AD	[18, 109, 110]
Axenfeld-Rieger syndrome type1 (180500)	PITX2	Brain abnormalities, variable pituitary deficiency	AD	[109]
Optic nerve hypoplasia and abnormalities of the central nervous system (206900)	SOX2	Variable GHD, LH and FSH deficiency, developmental delay	AD	[109, 110]
X-linked panhypopituitarism (312000, 300123)	SOX3	GHD or CPHD, mental retardation	XLR	[18, 109, 110]
Pellister-Hall syndrome (146510)	FGF8	Holoprosencephaly, septo-optic dysplasia, Moebius syndrome	AR	[18, 110]
	FGFR1	Pituitary and corpus callosum hypoplasia, ocular defects	AD	[18, 111]
	PROKR2	Variable pituitary hormone deficiency	AD	[111]

*Name (number) according to OMIM.

Abbreviations: AD, autosomal dominant; AR, autosomal recessive; XLR, X-linked recessive.

Table 2. Genetic defects reported in CPHD.

3. Diagnosis of GHD

The diagnosis of GHD in children should be based on clinical and auxological assessment, and radiological evaluation, along with biochemical tests for the pituitary-IGF axis. In some cases, genetic testing is requested.

3.1. Clinical and auxological assessment

Growth hormone deficiency can develop at any age (from the first few months of life to adolescence) and signs may vary. Generally, the neonate with isolated GHD exhibits hypoglycemia, prolonged jaundice and microphallus and/or cryptorchidism in males [4].

In pre-pubertal short children, the most common symptoms of idiopathic GHD are short stature and reduced growth velocity for age. The phenotypic characteristic features of severe GHD are immature faces, prominent forehead, depressed midline development, single central incisor, optic nerve hypoplasia, thin and sparse hair, slow nail growth, high-pitched voice, low muscle bulk, increased subcutaneous fat and low-density lipoprotein cholesterol [4].

When GHD is suspected in a child with short stature, other causes of growth failure such as hypothyroidism, chronic systemic diseases, Turner syndrome, malnutrition or skeletal disorders should first be excluded before starting endocrinological evaluation.

As recommended by the Consensus Guidelines for Diagnosis and Treatment of GHD in Childhood and Adolescence from the 2000 meeting of the GH Research Society [21], statement criteria to start evaluation for GHD are as follows:

- Severe short stature (height <3 SD below the mean);
- Height less than -1.5 SD below the mid-parental height;
- Height less than -2 SD below mean and either height velocity less than -1 SD below mean over the past year or decrease in height SD of more than 0.5 SD over the past year;
- In the absence of short stature, height velocity less than -2 SD below mean over 1 year or less than -1.5 SD below mean over 2 years;
- Signs of intracranial lesion;
- Signs of combined pituitary hormone deficiency; and
- Neonatal signs and symptoms of GHD, including hypoglycaemia, prolonged jaundice, microphallus and/or cryptorchidism, cranial midline abnormalities.

Generally, children with GHD do not show any metabolic abnormalities, notwithstanding the biological effects of GH on the different metabolisms. Recently, we reported that lipid and glucose metabolism are only slightly affected in GHD children but GH replacement therapy affects the secretion of factors such as leptin and resistin by adipose tissue [22]. Growth-hormone-deficient patients frequently show reduced bone mineralization with decreased bone density for delayed skeletal maturation. However, a study by Hogler and collaborators demonstrated that, in GHD children, cortical and trabecular densities are normal and the risk of fracture is not increased [23]. Similarly, inflammatory cytokines, such as TNF-α, IL-6 and IL-12, are comparable between GHD children and age-matched healthy controls and are slightly influenced by a short-term rhGH therapy [24, 25].

3.2. Radiological investigations

In the child over 1 year of age, bone age is routinely estimated from an x-ray of the left wrist and hand [21]. Sometimes in 2- or 3-year-old children the results may not be accurate, bone age can be evaluated more precisely from X-rays of the knee and foot, as in the neonate. Generally, the severity and duration of GHD affects delayed bone maturation. Bone age is usually assessed using the Greulich and Pyle radiological atlas [26] and/or the Tanner and Whitehouse (the TW2) method [27].

Magnetic resonance imaging is the most frequently used technique to visualize hypothalamic-pituitary anatomy. Neuroimaging in short children may rule out a tumour, in particular a craniopharyngioma or optic nerve glioma. The most common radiological findings in GHD children are an ectopic posterior pituitary gland, anterior pituitary hypoplasia and a thin pituitary stalk, which may be also present in combination. Other abnormalities associated with GHD may be septo-optic dysplasia, corpus callosum hypoplasia and presence of empty sella. However, many idiopathic GHD children show no pituitary abnormalities and some authors demonstrated that those GHD children with MRI abnormalities have more severe short stature and younger age at diagnosis compared with those GHD patients with normal pituitary [28].

3.3. Provocative GH testing

The measurement of GH secretion and not of basal GH levels, which are normally low, is used for confirming the diagnosis of GHD. Growth hormone secretion is pulsatile throughout the 24 hours, with peaks occurring at the time of slow-wave electroencephalographic rhythm and is regulated by multiple peptides and neurotransmitters, in particular GHRH and somatostatin. Furthermore, GH secretion significantly varies with gender, age, weight and pubertal status: during puberty it markedly increases, due to increased sex steroid levels, and then it decreases with age, especially in males [29].

Different cut-off values in children, adolescents and adults have been proposed by the GH Research Society to confirm the diagnosis of GHD. However, a specific cut-off value based on age, sex, weight and pubertal stage does not exist and should be established to improve the interpretation of GH stimulation tests.

Therefore, in current clinical practice, the diagnosis of GHD relies on biochemical measurement of GH secretion after stimulation tests. Various commercially available assays for measuring GH exist and several studies have shown an inter-assay variability of GH values [30, 31] that leads to a wide discrepancy in the results obtained in different analysis laboratories. They remarkably depend on different factors, such as the assay methods and the different calibrators used, the specificity of antibodies (monoclonal or polyclonal), the matrix difference between standards and samples and the interference with endogenous GH binding proteins (GHBPs) [32].

Commercially available immunoassays may detect different GH variants present in serum, since GH circulates in many isoforms due to alternative splicing, polymerisation and complexing with other molecules [33]. Moreover, we recently reported that GH values may also depend on different calibrators (i.e. IS 98/574, a recombinant 22 kDa molecule of more than 95% purity, and IS 80/505, of pituitary origin and resembling a variety of GH isoforms) used in the same GH assay [34]. Variations in GHBP have been found to significantly affect the GH concentration detected, since in serum up to 50% of GH is bound to GHBP [35]. According to the most recent international recommendations on GH assay standardization, only the 22 kDa recombinant IS 98/574 should be used and GH results should be expressed in mass units and, since 2006, major clinical endocrinology journals accept only those manuscripts in which GH data are expressed in micrograms per litre for IS 98/574 [36, 37].

The effect of the assay variability can lead to significant differences in the diagnosis of GHD among laboratories, since different cut-off values are used. In fact, the serum GH cut-off value for GH secretion depends on the method used for determining serum GH [38]. Different immunoassays (RIA, IRMA, ELISA, chemiluminescent and immunofunctional assays) are widely used in clinical laboratories because of speed, sensitivity and convenience. However, cut-off limits of GH stimulation tests to diagnose GHD in childhood and adolescence are not sufficiently validated by clinical studies. In the last years, in clinical practice, the traditional cut-off value of 10 ng/ml, which had been validated in the 1960s and 1970s, using developed radioimmunoassay, was widely used [21]. Recently, a study by Wagner et al. established new method-specific clinical evidence-based GH cut-off limits, showing that those limits varied from 4.32 to 7.77 ng/ml for seven hGH assays [39]. Thus, the cut-off level for the diagnosis of GHD has been revised and 8 ng/ml is accepted as the cut-off limit using Immulite 2000 assay. A GH peak concentration below 4 ng/ml defines complete GHD and a peak between 4 and 8 ng/ml indicates partial GHD.

Furthermore, different cut-off points have been proposed based on children BMI and in response to GHRH+arginine test: for lean children a peak cut-off value of 11.5 ng/ml, for overweight children a peak cut-off value of 8 ng/ml and for obese children a peak cut-off value of 4.2 ng/ml [31]. However, these cut-off points have not yet been validated.

The consensus guidelines of the Growth Hormone Research Society for diagnosis and treatment of GHD in children have established that in a child with suspected isolated GHD, two stimulation tests are required, since there are large numbers of false positive diagnoses from single stimulation test in normal children [21]. On the contrary, in a child with central nervous system pathology, cranial irradiation or genetic defects only one GH stimulation test is needed [21]. Due to the lack of reproducibility and accuracy of these tests, the clinician should remember that the diagnosis of GHD is mainly based on clinical and auxological findings and that the results of the stimulation tests are only confirmatory [40].

Many different stimuli are currently used to induce GH secretion, since they act through different mechanisms. Indeed, no stimulation test is completely reliable, although for clinical practice the Insulin Tolerance Test (ITT) is the gold standard [29]. As summarized in **Table 3**, different pharmacological stimuli are used to measure GH secretion [41]. Sometimes, to improve specificity of the test, pharmacological stimuli may be combined, for example, the combination of GHRH and arginine. These tests should be carefully monitored by an experienced team.

Stimulus	Dosage	Time samples (minutes)
Insulin tolerance test i.v.	0.05–0.01 U/kg	0, 15, 30, 45, 60 and 90
Arginine HCl i.v.	0.5 g/kg (max 40 g)	0, 30, 60, 90 and 120
Clonidine i.v.	0.15 mg/m^2	0, 30, 60 and 90
Glucagon i.m.	0.03 mg/kg (max 1 mg)	0, 30, 60, 90, 120, 150 and 180
GHRH i.v.+arginine HCl i.v.	1 μg/kg GHRH, arginine 0.5 g/kg (maximum of 40 g)	0, 15, 30, 45, 60, 90 and 120

i.v., intravenously; i.m., intramuscularly; p.o., per os.

Table 3. Currently used GH stimulation tests.

Insulin tolerance test is considered the best stimulation test, although it is risky because of the hypoglycaemia induced by insulin administration. GH secretion is stimulated by the response to insulin-induced hypoglycaemia. Usually, 0.1 unit/kg of insulin is administered intravenously (i.v.) in children over 4 years of age and 0.05 unit/kg in younger children. Blood samples for GH analysis and glucose levels should be obtained at 0, 15, 30, 45, 60 and 90 minutes after administering the insulin dose. The test is considered valid if the blood glucose level decreases by 40–50% of the initial value or reaches less than 40 mg/dl (i.e. 2.22 mmol/l). The GH peak occurs 15–30 minutes after the glucose nadir. Children with GHD frequently have an enhanced response to insulin that results in severe hypoglycaemia.

Arginine stimulates GH secretion by inhibition of somatostatin release. Arginine HCl (0.5 g/kg to a maximum of 40 g) is administered i.v. over a 30-minute period. Blood samples for GH determination should be taken at 0 (baseline), 30, 60, 90 and 120 minutes. The maximum GH peak is expected to occur at 60 minutes after starting arginine infusion. Nausea and vomiting are frequently observed side effects.

Clonidine, an alpha 2-adrenergic agonist, increases GHRH secretion and inhibits somatostatin release. Clonidine is administered at a dose of 0.15 mg/m^2 [42]. Samples for this GH assay should be obtained at 0 (baseline), 30, 60 and 90 minutes. GH peak is usually recorded 60 minutes after clonidine administration and is usually greater than in tests with other stimuli. After clonidine administration, blood pressure may fall, and young children may show drowsiness for several hours.

Glucagone is another very used stimuli for GH secretion, which is stimulated by endogenous insulin glucagon-induced to compensate for elevated serum glucose levels. Glucagon is administered intramuscularly (i.m.) or subcutaneously (s.c.) at a dose of 0.03 mg/kg to a maximum of 1 mg. Serum samples are obtained at 0, 30, 60, 90, 120, 150 and 180 minutes after administration. The maximal GH peak can occur 2 hours after glucagon injection. After glucagon administration young children may develop nausea and vomit.

Growth hormone releasing hormone is the endogenous stimulating factor of GH and the administration of GHRH can directly assess the capacity of the pituitary to secrete GH. Somatostatin inhibitors, pyridostigmine and arginine are used to enhance the GH response and to reduce the intra- and inter-individual variability, due to fluctuations in somatostatin secretion. The GHRH test, in combination with arginine, is a very useful tool to identify defects at the hypothalamic level, especially in children with CPHD. The GHRH+arginine test stimulates GH to a greater extent than the GHRH test alone. Growth hormone releasing hormone is given i.v. at a dose of 1 μg/kg at time 0 and arginine, at a dose of 0.5 g/kg (maximum of 40 g), i.v. infusion is given from time 0 to time 30. Serum samples for the GH analysis are obtained at 0, 15, 30, 45, 60, 90 and 120 minutes. The cut-off for this test is 20 ng/ml for the GH peak in childhood and 19.0 ng/ml in late adolescent and early adulthood [43]. Furthermore, the GHRH plus arginine test is useful for identifying false positive GHD in children showing a blunted GH response to classic stimuli in contrast with a normal growth rate [44]. Finally, GHRH+arginine test is particularly used in the re-testing of GH secretion at the end of GH therapy in childhood-onset GHD patients.

Growth hormone secretion may be evaluated by more physiologic tests, such as the exercise test, 24-h GH profiling and urinary GH estimation. Although they show minimal side effects for the patient and are less expensive than pharmacological tests, these tests are no longer used for the diagnosis of GHD in clinical practice, but they are still useful for research investigation.

GH testing in children in the peri-pubertal period and in those with delayed puberty frequently yields subnormal results due to a diagnosis of constitutional delay or, more probably, a sex steroid deficiency, since circulating levels of sex steroids increase during puberty, resulting in an increase in pulse amplitude of GH secretion, IGF-I concentration and anterior pituitary size. Therefore, the use of oestrogen or testosterone to prime the GH axis prior to pharmacological stimulation tests may facilitate GH release in pre-pubertal children and reduce false positive rates. Priming may be performed with oral oestrogen (10–20 μg ethinyloestradiol) for 3 days prior to GH stimulation test in girls or intramuscular injection of testosterone enanthate (100 mg) 7–10 days prior to stimulation test in boys [3]. However, not all paediatric endocrinologists agree that sex-hormone priming is required [45], since it only briefly augments the GH response which then returns to suboptimal concentrations and this may lead to under-diagnosis of peri-pubertal children that could have benefited from GH treatment. Some authors recommend that priming may be considered only in adolescents with pubertal delay (girls aged >11.5–12 years and boys aged >13–13.5 years) with no signs of puberty or only initial ones [46]. Therefore, at present there is no agreement on the use of priming.

3.4. Measurement of IGF-I and IGFBP-3

Because of the low reliability of the pharmacological tests, in the last years newer diagnostic procedures such as assay of IGF-I and IGFBP-3 serum levels, genetic testing and neuroimaging have been considered for confirming the diagnosis of GHD in children [47]. However, in many European countries it is yet mandatory to show a reduced GH secretion to at least two stimulation tests in order to start substitutive rhGH therapy in children.

The IGFs are GH-dependent peptides that mediate many of the anabolic and mitogenic actions of GH. The levels of IGF-I and its major binding protein IGFBP-3 greatly depend on GH secretion. Since serum levels of IGF-I are stable during the day, it should be possible to assess GH status by measuring IGF-I levels. However, most of the assays for IGF-I measurements do not show good sensitivity and specificity and are used in the diagnosis of GHD in children [48]. Furthermore, since IGF-I levels are influenced by age and pubertal development, an overlap between IGF-I values for normal and GHD children still exists, particularly in children younger than 5 years. Most investigators use cut-offs of either the fifth percentile or <-2 SD score to define subnormal levels of IGF-I [47]. Moreover, reduced IGF-I levels may occur in children with malnutrition, hypothyroidism, hepatic disease or diabetes mellitus.

Insulin-like growth factor binding protein-3 levels have also been considered for the detection of GHD and were thought to be potentially superior to measurement of IGF-I alone as IGFBP-3 is less nutritionally sensitive than IGF-I. However, many studies found no differences in IGFBP-3 levels between GHD and non-GHD subjects [49].

In conclusion, although reduced IGF-I and IGFBP-3 levels may suggest a condition of severe GHD, normal serum IGF-I and IGFBP-3 values may not allow to exclude GHD. Therefore, GH stimulation tests are widely used for confirming GHD diagnosis in children.

3.5. Genetic investigation

Genetic testing is not routinely performed in the diagnosis of GHD. However, numerous mutations leading to GHD have been identified and with the development of new genetic technologies, such as whole exome and whole genome sequencing, screening for mutations in the diagnosis of GHD may play a critical role in the coming years.

Generally, signs of GHD of genetic origin are particularly evident and may include: early onset of growth failure, positive family history, height more than 3 SD below the mean, extremely low GH response to provocation tests, very low IGF-I and IGFBP-3 levels. In these cases, genetic analysis is strongly suggested.

The most common mutations in patients with isolated GHD have been identified in *GH1*, *GHRHR* and *RNPC3* genes and may be associated with a normal MRI scan (**Table 1**). Other gene mutations (i.e. *POU1F1*, *PROP1*, *LHX3*, *LHX4*, *HESX1*, *SOX2*, *SOX3*, etc.) present in GHD, along with other pituitary deficiency, are associated with clinical and radiological features (**Table 2**).

4. Treatment of GHD children

As recommended by the GH Research Society [21], patients with proven GHD should be treated with rhGH as soon as possible after the diagnosis is made, for normalizing height during childhood and obtaining normal adult height. The response to GH therapy could be affected by variables such as birth-weight, age and height at start of treatment and at start of puberty, extent of the GHD and duration of treatment [50, 51]. The pattern of catch-up growth in GHD infants during GH therapy indicates a sustained and significant effect during the first years of treatment, followed by a progressive decrease in growth velocity, known as "waning effect" in the subsequent years [52]. Nevertheless, the growth rate is always higher than it was before starting the therapy, suggesting that GH therapy may still be advantageous for patients.

Growth hormone treatment in childhood also normalizes body composition, reducing body fat, generating a reversible insulin insensitivity, increasing the ratio of high-density lipoprotein to total cholesterol and accelerating bone remodelling with the increase of bone mineral mass [22].

Until 1985, for more than 30 years, GHD was treated by pituitary-derived GH. Then, rhGH was introduced into clinical practice and now the presently available rhGH brands for registered clinical indications are obtained by expression either in *Escherichia coli* bacteria or in mammalian cell lines, such as mouse C127. Recently, identical recombinant DNA-derived proteins have been expressed in other biological systems (i.e. *Saccharomyces cerevisiae*); these proteins have the same structure and similar profiles in terms of quality, safety and efficacy and are termed "biosimilars."

Growth hormone should be administered s.c. in the evening on a daily basis, and the rhGH dosage should be expressed in milligrams per kilogram of body weight per day. The recommended starting dosage for rhGH is 0.025–0.05 mg/kg/day, according to a 6-day per week schedule. An increment in the dose from 0.03 to 0.07 mg/kg per day is suggested during puberty, to maximize longitudinal growth during this period of life. An alternative approach to the fixed dose is auxology-based dosing. This approach consists of starting treatment with the lowest accepted dose and then titrating upwards based on weight, growth velocity and IGF-I concentrations, still keeping the GH dose within the dose range [53]. IGF-I titration consists in adjusting the GH dose to a target IGF-I concentration irrespective of growth rate and the usual range of GH dose. This leads to the use of very high GH doses (i.e. 0.091 mg/kg/day) in order to find an improvement in growth rate in comparison with patients treated with a fixed dose [54]. Since there are very few safety data on the use of GH at such high doses, this approach cannot be recommended at the present time. Actually, the major current alternative strategy is prediction model-based dosing. Prediction models may lead to a more evidence-based approach to determine the GH dose regimen and may reduce the response variability and drug costs for GH treatment. Three types of prediction models have been described, all using auxological data. It is uncertain whether adding biochemical, genetic or proteomic markers may improve the accuracy of the prediction [55].

Subcutaneous injection (s.c.) has become the standard administration route for GH because of its ease of administration and patient acceptance. Among experimental studies on possible other ways of delivery of GH, a multi-centre study focused its attention on the inhalator route [56]. The authors showed that GH delivered by inhalation was well tolerated and resulted in a dose-dependent increase in serum GH and IGF-I levels, suggesting that the delivery of GH via the deep lung is feasible in children and should deserve attention.

Furthermore, in order to obtain a better compliance of patients to years of daily treatment, long-acting forms of GH have been developed, utilizing different techniques: depot GH formulations, pegylated formulations, pro-drug formulations and GH fusion protein technology [57]. These formulations show different pharmacodynamic and pharmacokinetic profiles, all being effective in extending GH action and prolonging increase IGF-I concentrations. Clinical data in humans are still very limited and short-term studies showed that treatment with long-acting GH preparation is effective and safe in GHD children and adults. Many of these formulations frequently showed injection-site reactions with erythema, induration or lipoatrophy. Long-term studies are needed to confirm the value and safety of these agents [58].

The routine follow-up of GHD children should be performed by a paediatric endocrinologist on a 3- to 6-month basis. The determination of the increase in height and change in height velocity during rhGH treatment is useful in assessing the response to GH. A study from the International Growth Study database (KIGS) showed that during GH therapy it is important to monitor IGF-I levels to check the compliance of the patients and ensure that IGF-I values do not exceed the normal range, since high levels of IGF-I have been linked to the development of tumours [59]. Therefore, supra-physiological concentrations of IGF-I should be avoided [60].

If GHD is part of a combined pituitary insufficiency, it is necessary to address each endocrine deficiency. Thyroid stimulating hormone deficiency is often unmasked during the initial phase of rhGH therapy. During the follow-up of GH therapy, every 6 months, FT4 and TSH should be evaluated and, if a decrease is observed, a TRH stimulation test should be performed. Patients with a deficit of ACTH should be placed on the lowest safe maintenance dose of glucocorticoids, no more than 10 mg/m^2 per day of hydrocortisone, since higher doses may impair the growth response to rhGH therapy. Gonadotropin deficiency may be evident in infancy in a child with microphallus. In patients with CPHD, it is appropriate to begin sex steroid replacement at an appropriate age, since physical and psychological benefits of normalizing sexual maturation must be balanced against the risk of epiphyseal fusion. Assessment of skeletal maturation is useful to prevent rapid epiphyseal closure and loss in adult height. In males, this can be done by beginning at 13–14 years of age with 50 mg testosterone enanthate i.m. every month for about 12 months. Over the next 3–4 years, the dose should gradually be increased to the adult replacement dose of 250 mg every 2–3 weeks. Transdermal testosterone patches and gels have recently become available, which may produce consistent serum levels of testosterone in older adolescents on a stable replacement dose. In girls, therapy involves the use of conjugated oestrogens or ethynil estradiol: low doses of ethinyl estradiol (20 μg) increased over the next 1–2 years, after which a progestin is added to the last 5–7 days of the cycle to induce bleeding. Once cycling has been induced, it is generally more convenient to use one of the oestrogen-progestin combination oral contraceptive pills [61]. In these patients, fertility is possible with the use of chorionic gonadotropin, human menotropins, GnRH agonist and other fertility medications. Patients also need to understand that gonadal steroid replacement therapy is necessary for the greater part of their adult life to maintain bone mineral density.

4.1. GH treatment of children after bone marrow transplantation (BMT) for acute leukaemia

Growth impairment and GHD have been frequently observed in children after BMT with TBI and those previously undergoing central nervous system irradiation to treat acute leukaemia [62]. These therapies may compromise growth pubertal development, and consequently final height. However, since the diagnosis of GHD in such patients is made shortly after the end of the irradiation, their growth rate may not be as decreased and their bone age as delayed as in idiopathic GHD children. In our previous paper [63], we showed growth rate impairment both in children who have received TBI and chemotherapy as a preparative regimen and in children receiving prophylactic cranial irradiation before being conditioned with TBI and chemotherapy (**Figure 1**). On the other hand, patients transplanted after a busulfan-containing myeloablative therapy did not experience significant problems in terms of growth velocity [63]. With the increasing number of survivors and duration of follow-up, patients may experience a significant loss of height potential and GH treatment may have beneficial effects. In our GH-treated patients, a successful response was observed with increase in growth rate during the first 2 years of therapy [63]. More recently, other authors found a measurable catch-up growth and a normalization of final height in patients timely treated with GH, thus reducing the

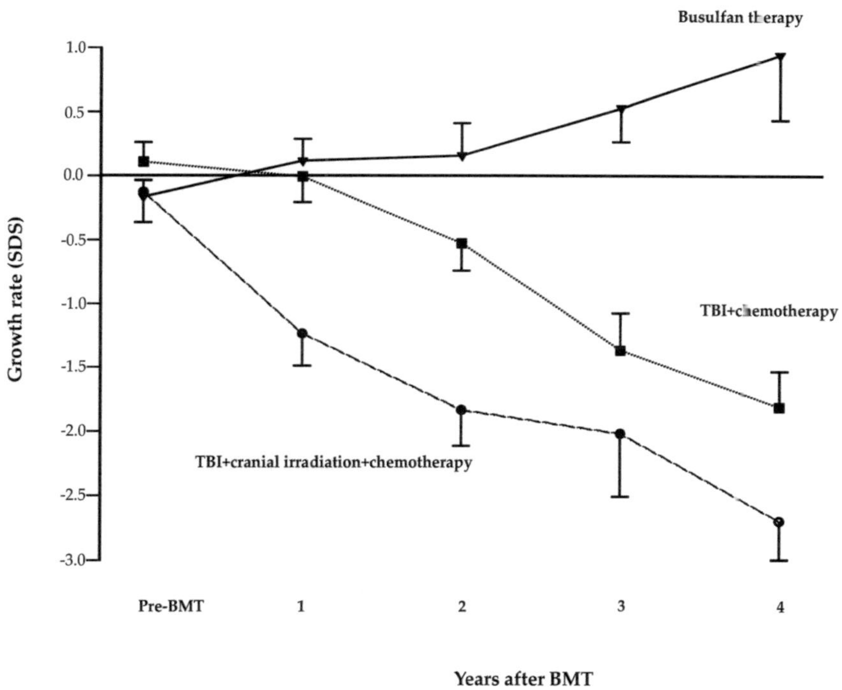

Figure 1. Mean growth rate SDS before and after BMT in the three groups of children with different conditioning regimens before transplantation [63]. Data are expressed as mean ± standard deviation.

negative impact of the acute leukaemia-related treatment on the growth of paediatric patients [64]. The dosages of GH used in these studies are not different from those used in idiopathic GHD children, ranging from 0.020 to 0.033 mg/kg body weight/day. However, clinicians should be aware that children with prior malignancies show an increase in oncologic risk, especially if treatment of the primary malignancy involved radiation therapy [65].

We therefore propose that all children treated with haematopoietic stem cell transplantation, TBI or central irradiation should routinely undergo, once a year, testing of GH secretion and endocrine evaluation. When GHD is biochemically proven, GH replacement therapy should be considered in order to ameliorate the final growth. However, patients with an active malignancy should not receive GH, and patients whose tumour is no longer active should be carefully monitored for any evidence of progression or recurrence.

4.2. Variability in the response to rhGH therapy

The catch-up growth in response to rhGH therapy is maximal during the first year and typically attenuates during the following years. However, growth velocity is still comparable to healthy age-matched children.

The first-year growth response depends on several factors including dose and frequency of administration and age at the start of rhGH treatment. The first-year growth response is inversely correlated with GH peak during stimulation test and age at the start of replacement therapy and is positively correlated with rhGH dose, weight at the start of replacement therapy and weight at birth. We recently reported that birth size is an important factor affecting the response to GH therapy in GHD children during the first 5 years of treatment. In fact, when GHD children showed small size for their gestational age a blunted response to GH therapy is observed, in comparison to GHD children born with an adequate size and weight for gestational age [66].

Furthermore, the first year growth response to GH may predict up to 7 years of pre-pubertal growth in GHD children and can be used as an aid-in-treatment decision making [67]. Patients with severe GHD show a better growth response in the first year of replacement therapy than those with moderate GHD. For the second, third and fourth years, growth responses are positively correlated with height velocity during the preceding year, weight and weekly rhGH dose, and negatively correlated with chronological age [68]. Recently, the authors of KIGS concluded that IGF-I monitoring during GH therapy is a valuable tool for evaluating compliance and may help clinicians change GH doses to achieve normal serum IGF-I and normal growth [69, 70].

Pharmacogenomic studies have showed that GH receptor (GHR) is the key molecule mediating GH action and that a GHR gene polymorphism (absence of exon 3, d3-GHR) has an influence on the response to rhGH therapy. However, the results of the numerous studies on this issue are still contradictory. Some studies demonstrated that GHD patients carrying the d3-GHR allele had a better response to substitutive GH therapy than patients with the normal allele [71–73], while other studies did not. This may be due to confounding factors such as small sample size, differences in experimental design and severity of GHD [74–78]. In fact, more recent results from the PREDICT Study demonstrated that response to rhGH depends on the interaction between GHD severity and d3-GHR carriage [79].

Although this d3-GHR genotype was the first identified genetic factor found to modulate the individual response to rhGH therapy, recently, other studies have shown that other polymorphisms of the GHR and of other molecules involved in GH/IGF-I axis (i.e. IGFBP-3 and SOCS2) could have a role in determining the response to rhGH therapy in GHD children [80–82]. These studies may better define the use of GHR polymorphism analysis in clinical practice, moving from pharmacogenetics to routine application and allowing individualization of rhGH doses to optimize final outcome.

4.3. Adherence to GH therapy

Since GH treatment requires regular, daily subcutaneous injections for very long periods, one of the primary causes of GH therapy failure is patient non-adherence to the prescribed drug therapy (daily injections missed or duration of the prescribed regimen not followed), especially in adolescents. No general consensus on the definition of good adherence has been reported and, therefore, the rate of non-adherence to paediatric GH therapy varies between 36% and 49% [83], depending on the detection methods and the definitions used. There is no gold standard method for measuring adherence; the methods most used are direct evaluation of drug levels or its metabolites (urinary GH or serum IGF-I), or indirect evaluation of prescription refills, clinical response, electronic devices or questionnaires completed by patients and/or their parents [84, 85]. Most of these methods are inconvenient for patients or imprecise, underscoring the difficulty for physicians to accurately assess the degree of adherence [86, 87]. The causes of non-adherence are often unknown and may be due to the different lifestyles of the patients, including socio-economic status, level of understanding and type of relationship with the child's physician. Other factors influencing adherence include the complexity of treatment regimens, the long-term nature of the therapy and the discomfort or pain associated with injections [83, 88]. In order to efficaciously improve adherence in GHD patients, appropriate pre-intervention discussion is essential, and should include a clear statement of the short- and long-term treatment targets. Carefully constructed healthcare plans are the key and should include educational programmes, home support and regular reinforcement. Furthermore, it is mandatory to regularly interview patients with a non-aggressive approach to ensure effective communication with patients and their parents [89].

4.4. Side effects of GH therapy

Overall, significant side effects of rhGH therapy in children and adolescents are very rare and include benign intracranial hypertension (frequency between 1/10,000 and 1/1000) and paraesthesia (between 1/1000 and 1/100), arthralgia and myalgia (between 1/100 and 1/10). Recombinant hGH treatment may represent a risk factor for type 2 diabetes in predisposed patients (frequency between 1/10,000 and 1/1000). In general, these events are exaggerated physiologic effects of rhGH (i.e. sodium and water retention, growth rate acceleration) or are due to underlying conditions in treated patients. Management of these side effects may include either a transient reduction of dosage or temporary discontinuation of GH therapy.

In conclusion, the side effects of GH treatment are uncommon in children and the treatment can be considered safe. Only in children with Prader-Willi syndrome treated with GH, have some cases of sudden death been reported due to obstructive sleep apnoea. In any case, these patients deserve particular attention and polysomnography monitoring and otorhinolaryngoiatric video endoscopy should be performed before and after beginning GH therapy [90].

The development of growth-inhibiting GH antibodies is extremely rare and limited to the IGHD IA form, although anti-GH antibodies without blocking activity have recently also been detected in a girl with idiopathic GHD [91]. Finally, there is no evidence that rhGH replacement needs to be discontinued during inter-current illness.

Considering the potential for side effects in the use of a growth promoting agent as GH, the community of physicians and pharmaceutical manufacturers have developed systematic methods to survey for short- and long-term effects. Recently, the Safety and Appropriateness of Growth Hormone treatments in Europe (SAGhE) study assembled the largest cohort of GH-treated patients with the longest follow-up for investigating cancer and mortality risks. Interestingly, the analysis was independent of industry. The preliminary results are, however, contrasting [92]. In fact, the French SAGhE has raised concerns of increased mortality risk due to bone tumours or cerebral haemorrhage during follow-up into adulthood, especially in patients who had received high GH doses during childhood [93]. On the contrary, a study on the cohorts from Sweden, Belgium and The Netherlands of the SAGhE reported no increased mortality. The authors showed that the majority of deaths (76%) were caused by accidents or suicides and, more importantly, none of the patients died from cancer or from a cardiovascular disease [94]. More recently, a sponsored observational study (The Hypopituitary Control and Complications Study, HypoCCS) confirmed no increased risk of mortality or incidence of cancer, stroke or myocardial infarction in adult GH-deficient patients who had previously received paediatric GH treatment [95]. These results stress the importance of studies of long-term outcomes after childhood treatments and highlight the need for similar studies to be performed elsewhere.

5. GH therapy in transition age

Growth hormone deficiency may or may not persist into adult life. Patients with childhood onset GHD are usually retested in late adolescence or young adulthood in order to confirm the GHD diagnosis. The 2007 Consensus guidelines for the diagnosis and treatment of GHD adults and its update in 2011 stated that in idiopathic GHD children a re-evaluation by GH stimulation tests is required, unless there is a proven genetic/structural lesion persistent from childhood [96, 97]. At this time, it is important to measure also IGF-I levels and secretion of other pituitary hormones. Re-evaluation of the GH status has shown that GHD is permanent in patients with CPHD, acquired hypothalamic-pituitary lesions, pituitary hypoplasia, pituitary stalk agenesis and posterior pituitary ectopia. On the contrary, a high proportion of children with isolated GHD and no pituitary abnormalities show a different percentage of normalization of GH secretion, ranging from 12.5% to 95% [98–101]. Our recently unpublished results showed that, at the time of re-testing, 82.1% of severe GHD and 82.4% of partial GHD patients showed transient GHD. This may be due to low reproducibility and high intra-individual variability of the stimulation tests used at the time of diagnosis. Furthermore, there are no clear data on normal GH values after GH stimulation and standardized cut-off levels available in adolescents and young adults. The Consensus guidelines recommended the use of the insulin tolerance test or GHRH+arginine test as provocative tests [97] for re-testing. However, these recommendations are based on limited existing evidence [102, 103] and should be further validated. Growth hormone therapy should be stopped at least 1 month before retesting, although a range of 1–3 months stop has been reported [104].

In the period from late adolescence to early adulthood, GH plays an important role in body composition regulation, muscle mass maturation, full skeletal mineralization and reproductive maturation, as well as in the prevention of metabolic and cardiovascular risk. Therefore, GH replacement should be restarted if a blunted GH secretion is still present [105]. The transition to adult rhGH replacement therapy should be arranged as a close collaboration between the paediatric and adult endocrinologists in order to determine the timing of the patient care transition and to minimize the interruption of GH therapy during the transition period.

Acknowledgements

The authors are grateful to Susan West for revising the English language of the paper.

Author details

Mauro Bozzola* and Cristina Meazza

*Address all correspondence to: mauro.bozzola@unipv.it

Internal Medicine and Therapeutics Department, Pediatrics and Adolescentology Unit, University of Pavia, Pavia, Italy

References

[1] Rogol AD, Hayden GF. Etiologies and early diagnosis of short stature and growth failure in children and adolescents. J Pediatr. 2014164:S1–S14.e6. DOI: 10.1016/j.jpeds.2014.02.027

[2] Allen DB, Cuttler L. Clinical practice. Short stature in childhood—challenges and choices. N Engl J Med. 2013;368:1220–1228. DOI: 10.1056/NEJMcp1213178

[3] Murray PG, Dattani MT, Clayton PE. Controviersies in the diagnosis and management of growth hormone deficiency in childhood and adolescence. Arch Dis Child. 2016;101:96–100. DOI: 10.1136/archdischild-2014-307228

[4] Reiter EO, Rosenfeld RG. Normal and aberrant growth. In: Kronenberg HM, Melmed S, Polonsky KS, Larsen PR, editors. Williams Textbook of Endocrinology (11th Edition). Philadelphia, USA: Saunders Elsevier, 2008; p. 849–968.

[5] Rappaport R, Bowlby DA. Clinical aspects of growth and growth disorders. In: Pescovitz OH and Eugster EA, editors. Pediatric Endocrinology. Mechanisms, Manifestations, and Management. Philadelphia, USA: Lippincott Williams & Wilkins, 2004; p. 178.

[6] Argente J. Challenges in the management of short stature. Horm Res Paediatr. 2016;85:2–10. DOI: 10.1159/000442350

[7] Bozzola M, Mengarda F, Sartirana P, Tatò L, Chaussain JL. Long-term follow-up evaluation of magnetic resonance imaging in the prognosis of permanent GH deficiency. Eur J Endocrinol. 2000;143:493–496. DOI: 10.1530/eje.0.1430493

[8] De Bellis A, Colao A, Tirelli G Ruocco G, Di Somma C, Battaglia M, Pane E, Bellastella G, Dello Iacovo A, Sinisi AA, Bizzarro A, Bellastella A. Autoimmunity as a possible cause of growth hormone deficiency. J Endocrinol Invest. 2008;1:1132–1134.

[9] Wit JM, Oostdijk W, Losekoot M, van Duyvenvoorde HA, Ruivenkamp CA, Kant SG. Mechanisms in endocrinology: novel genetic causes of short stature. Eur J Endocrinol. 2016;174:R145–R173. DOI: 10.1530/EJE-15-0937

[10] Petkovic V, Godi M, Pandey AV, Lochmatter D, Buchanan CR, Dattani MT, Eble A, Fluck CE, Mullis PE. Growth hormone (GH) deficiency type II: a novel GH-1 gene mutation (GH-R178H) affecting secretion and action. J Clin Endocrinol Metab. 2010;95:731–739. DOI: 10.1210/jc.2009-1247

[11] Duriez B, Duquesnoy P, Dastot F, Bougneres P, Amselem S, Goossens M. An exon-skipping mutation in the btk gene of a patient with X-linked agammaglobulinemia and isolated growth hormone deficiency. FEBS Lett. 1994;346:165–170. DOI: 10.1016/0014-5793(94)00457-9

[12] Burkitt WEM, Perveen R, Clayton PE, Hall CM, Costa T, Procter AM, Giblin CA, Donnai D, Black GC. X-linked isolated growth hormone deficiency: expanding the phenotypic spectrum of SOX3 polyalanine tract expansions. Clin Dysmorphol. 2009;720:218–221. DOI: 10.1097/MCD.0b013e32832d06f0

[13] Wit JM, Oostdijk W, Losekoot M. Spectrum of insulin-like growth factor deficiency. Endocr Dev. 2012;23:30–41. DOI: 10.1159/000341739

[14] Argente J, Flores R, Gutierrez-Arumi A, Verma B, Martos-Moreno GA, Cusco I, Oghabian A, Chowen JA, Frilander MJ, Perez-Jurado LA. Defective

minor spliceosome mRNA processing results in isolated familial growth hormone deficiency. EMBO Mol Med. 2014;6:299–306. DOI: 10.1002/emmm.201303573

[15] Lucas-Herald AK, Kinning E, Iida A, Wang Z, Miyake N, Ikegawa S, McNeilly J, Ahmed SF. A case of functional growth hormone deficiency and early growth retardation in a child with IFT172 mutations. J Clin Endocrinol Metab. 2015;100:1221–1224. DOI: 10.1210/jc.2014-3852

[16] Romano S, Maffei P, Bettini V, Milan G, Favaretto F, Gardiman M, Marshall JD, Greggio NA, Pozzan GB, Collin GB, Naggert JK, Bronson R, Vettor R. Alstrom syndrome is associated with short stature and reduced GH reserve. Clin Endocrinol (Oxf). 2013;79:529–536. DOI: 10.1111/cen.12180

[17] Castinetti F, Reynaud R, Quentien MH, Jullien N, Marquant E, Rochette C, Herman JP, Saveanu A, Barlier A, Enjalbert A, Brue T. Combined pituitary hormone deficiency: current and future status. J Endocrinol Invest. 2015;38:1–12. DOI: 10.1007/s40618-014-0141-2

[18] Dauber A, Rosenfeld RG, Hirschhorn JN. Genetic evaluation of short stature. J Clin Endocrinol Metab. 2014;99:3080–3092. DOI: 10.1210/jc.2014-1506

[19] Pfäffle RW, Parks JS, Brown MR, Heimann G. Pit-1 and pituitary function. J Pediatr Endocrinol. 1993;6:229–233.

[20] Giordano M, Gertosio C, Pagani S, Meazza C, Fusco I, Bozzola E, Bozzola M. A 5.8 Mb interstitial deletion on chromosome Xq21.1 in a boy with intellectual disability, cleft palate, hearing impairment and combined growth hormone deficiency. BMC Med Genet. 2015;16:74. DOI: 10.1186/s12881-015-0220-z

[21] GH Research Society. Consensus guidelines for the diagnosis and treatment of growth hormone (GH) deficiency in childhood and adolescence: summary statement of the GH Research Society. J Clin Endocrinol Metab. 2000;85:3990–3993. DOI: http://dx.doi.org/10.1210/jcem.85.11.6984

[22] Meazza C, Elsedfy HH, Pagani S, Bozzola E, El Kholy M, Bozzola M. Metabolic parameters and adipokine profile in growth hormone deficient (GHD) children before and after 12-month GH treatment. Horm Metab Res. 2014;46:219–223. DOI: 10.1055/s-0033-1358730

[23] Högler W, Shaw N. Childhood growth hormone deficiency, bone density, structures and fractures: scrutinizing the evidence. Clin Endocrinol (Oxf). 2010;72:281–289. DOI: 10.1111/j.1365-2265.2009.03686.x

[24] Pagani S, Meazza C, Travaglino P, Moretta A, Bozzola M. Effect of growth hormone therapy on the proinflammatory cytokine profile in growth hormone-deficient children. Eur Cytokine Netw. 2005;16:65–69.

[25] Pagani S, Meazza C, Travaglino P, De Benedetti F, Tinelli C, Bozzola M. Serum cytokine levels in GH-deficient children during substitutive GH therapy. Eur J Endocrinol. 2005;152:207–210. DOI: 10.1530/eje.1.01827

[26] Greulich WW, Pyle SI. Radiographic Atlas of Skeletal Development of the Hand and Wrist (2nd Edition). Stanford, USA: Stanford University Press, 1959.

[27] Tanner JM, Whitehouse RH, Cameron N, Marshall WA, Healy MJR, Godstein H. Assessment of Skeletal Maturation and Prediction of Adult Height (TW2 Method). New York, USA: New York Academic Press, 1983.

[28] Coutant R, Rouleau S, Despert F, Magontier N, Loisel D, Limal JM. Growth and adult height in GH-treated children with nonacquired GH deficiency and idiopathic short stature: the influence of pituitary magnetic resonance imaging findings. J Clin Endocrinol Metab. 2001;86:4649–4654.

[29] Richmond EJ, Rogol AD. Growth hormone deficiency in children. Pituitary. 2008;11:115–120. DOI: 10.1007/s11102-008-0105-7

[30] Chaler EA, Rivarola MA, Guerci B Ciaccio M, Costanzo M, Travaglino P, Maceiras M, Pagani S, Meazza C, Bozzola E, Barberi S, Bozzola M, Belgorosky A. Differences in serum GH cut-off values for pharmacological tests of GH secretion depend on the serum GH method. Clinical validation from the growth velocity score during the first year of treatment. Horm Res. 2006;66:231–235. DOI: 10.1159/000095005

[31] Corneli G, Di Somma C, Baldelli R, Rovere S, Gasco V, Croce CG, Grottoli S, Maccario M, Colao A, Lombardi G, Ghigo E, Camanni F, Aimaretti G. The cut-off limits of the GH response to GH-releasing hormone-arginine test related to body mass index. Eur J Endocrinol. 2005;153:257–264. DOI: 10.1530/eje.1.01967

[32] Clemmons DR. Consensus statement on the standardization and evaluation of growth hormone and insulin-like growth factor assays. Clin Chem 2011;57:555–559. DOI: 10.1373/clinchem.2010

[33] Baumann G. Growth hormone heterogeneity: genes, isohormones, variants and binding proteins. Endocr Rev. 1991;12:424–429. DOI: http://dx.doi.org/10.1210/edrv-12-4-424#sthash.GG0TtIoU.dpuf

[34] Meazza C, Albertini R, Pagani S, Sessa N, Laarej K, Falcone R, Bozzola E, Calcaterra V, Bozzola M. Diagnosis of growth hormone deficiency is affected by calibrators used in GH immunoassays. Horm Metab Res. 2012;44:900–903. DOI: 10.1055/s-0032-1314855

[35] Ebdrup L, Fisker S, Sørensen HH, Ranke MB, Orskov H. Variety in growth hormone determinations due to use of different immunoassays and to the interference of growth hormone-binding protein. Horm Res. 1999;51:20–26. DOI:10.1159/000053131

[36] Trainer PJ, Barth J, Sturgeon C, Wieringaon G. Consensus statement on the standardisation of GH assays. Eur J Endocrinol. 2006;155:1–2. DOI: 10.1530/eje.1.02186

[37] Sheppard MC. Growth hormone assay standardization: an important clinical advance. Clin Endocrinol (Oxf). 2007;66:157–161. DOI: 10.1111/j.1365-2265.2007.02703.x

[38] Popii V, Baumann G. Laboratory measurement of growth hormone. Clin Chim Acta. 2004;350:1–16. DOI: 10.1016/j.cccn.2004.06.007

[39] Wagner IV, Paetzold C, Gausche R, Vogel M, Koerner A, Thiery J, Arsene CG, Henrion A, Guettler B, Keller E, Kiess W, Pfaeffle R, Kratzsch J. Clinical evidence-based cutoff limits for GH stimulation tests in children with a backup of results with reference to mass spectrometry. Eur J Endocrinol. 2014;171:389–397. DOI: 10.1530/EJE-14-0165

[40] Hilczer M, Smyczynska J, Stawerska R, Lewinski A. Stability of IGF-I concentration despite divergent results of repeated GH stimulating tests indicates poor reproducibility of test results. Endocr Regul. 2006;40:37–45.

[41] Bozzola M, Meazza C. Growth hormone deficiency: diagnosis and therapy in children. Expert Rev Endocrinol Metab. 2010;2:273–284. DOI: 10.1586/eem.09.69

[42] Gil-Ad I, Topper E, Laron Z. Oral clonidine as a growth hormone stimulation test. Lancet. 1979;2:278–279. DOI: 10.1016/S0140-6736(79)90293-9

[43] Gasco V, Corneli G, Beccuti G, Prodam F, Rovere S, Bellone J, Grottoli S, Aimaretti G, Ghigo E. Retesting the childhood-onset GH-deficient patient. Eur J Endocrinol. 2008;159:S45–S52. DOI: 10.1530/EJE-08-0293

[44] Mazzola A, Meazza C, Travaglino P, Pagani S, Frattini D, Bozzola E, Corneli G, Aimaretti G, Bozzola M. Unreliability of classic provocative tests for the diagnosis of growth hormone deficiency. J Endocrinol Invest. 2008;31:159–162. DOI: 10.1007/BF03345583

[45] Molina S, Paoli M, Camacho N, Arata-Bellabarba G, Lanes R. Is testosterone and estrogen priming prior to clonidine useful in the evaluation of the growth hormone status of short peripubertal children? J Pediatr Endocrinol Metab. 2008;21:257–266. DOI: 10.1515/JPEM.2008.21.3.257

[46] Lazar L, Phillip M. Is sex hormone priming in peripubertal children prior to growth hormone stimulation tests still appropriate? Horm Res Paediatr. 2010;73:299–302. DOI: 10.1159/000284396

[47] Badaru A, Wilson DM. Alternatives to growth hormone stimulation testing in children. Trends Endocrinol Metab. 2004;15:252–258. DOI: 10.1016/j.tem.2004.06.004

[48] Obara-Moszyńska M, Kedzia A, Korman E, Niedziela M. Usefulness of growth hormone (GH) stimulation tests and IGF-I concentration measurement in GH deficiency diagnosis. J Pediatr Endocrinol Metab. 2008;21:569–579.

[49] Phillip M, Chalew SA, Kowarski AA, Stene MA. Plasma IGFBP-3 and its relationship with quantitative growth hormone secretion in short children. Clin Endocrinol (Oxf). 1993;39:427–432. DOI: 10.1111/j.1365-2265.1993.tb02389.x

[50] Blethen SL, Baptista J, Kuntze J, Foley T, LaFranchi S, Johanson A. Adult height in growth hormone (GH)-deficient children treated with biosynthetic GH. The Genentech Growth Study Group. J Clin Endocrinol Metab. 1997;82:418–420.

[51] Rappaport R, Mugnier E, Limoni C, Crosnier H, Czernichow P, Leger J, Limal JM, Rochiccioli P, Soskin S. A 5-year prospective study of growth hormone (GH)-deficient children treated with GH before the age of 3 years. J Clin Endocrinol Metab. 1997;82:452–456. DOI: http://dx.doi.org/10.1210/jcem.82.2.3756

[52] Frasier SD. Human pituitary growth hormone (hGH) therapy in growth hormone deficiency. Endocr Rev. 1983;4:155–170. DOI: http://dx.doi.org/10.1210/edrv-4-2-155

[53] Cutfield WS, Lundgren F. Insulin-like growth factor I and growth responses during the first year of growth hormone treatment in KIGS patients with idiopathic growth hormone deficiency, acquired growth hormone deficiency, turner syndrome and born small for gestational age. Horm Res. 2009;71:39–45. DOI: 10.1159/000178036

[54] Cohen P, Germak J, Rogol AD, Weng W, Kappelgaard AM, Rosenfeld RG; American Norditropin Study Group. Variable degree of growth hormone (GH) and insulin-like growth factor (IGF) sensitivity in children with idiopathic short stature compared with GH-deficient patients: evidence from an IGF-based dosing study of short children. J Clin Endocrinol Metab. 2010;95:2089–2098. DOI: 10.1210/jc.2009-2139

[55] Wit JM, Ranke MB, Albertsson-Wikland K, Carrascosa A, Rosenfeld RG, Van Buuren S, Kristrom B, Schoenau E, Audi L, Hokken-Koelega AC, Bang P, Jung H, Blum WF, Silverman LA, Cohen P, Cianfarani S, Deal C, Clayton PE, de Graaff L, Dahlgren J, Kleintjens J, Roelants M. Personalized approach to growth hormone treatment: clinical use of growth prediction models. Horm Res Paediatr. 2013;79:257–270. DOI: 10.1159/000351025

[56] Walvoord EC, de la Peña A, Park S, Silverman B, Cuttler L, Rose SR, Cutler G, Drop S, Chipman J. Inhaled growth hormone (GH) compared with subcutaneous GH in children with GH deficiency: pharmacokinetics, pharmacodynamics, and safety. J Clin Endocrinol Metab. 2009;94:2052–2059. DOI: 10.1210/jc.2008-1897

[57] Høybye C, Cohen P, Hoffman AR, Ross R, Biller BM, Christiansen JS; Growth Hormone Research Society. Status of long-acting-growth hormone preparations--2015. Growth Horm IGF Res. 2015;25:201–206. DOI: 10.1016/j.ghir.2015.07.004

[58] Doknic M, Stojanovic M, Popovic V. Novel long-acting GH preparations. Pediatr Endocrinol Rev. 2014;12:206–212.

[59] Park P, Cohen P. The role of insulin-like growth factor I monitoring in growth hormone-treated children. Horm Res. 2004;62:59–65. DOI: 10.1159/000080760

[60] Höybye C, Christiansen JS. Growth hormone replacement in adults—current standards and new perspectives. Best Pract Res Clin Endocrinol Metab. 2015;29:115–123. DOI: 10.1016/j.beem.2014.09.006

[61] Styne DM, Grumbach M. Puberty: ontogeny, neuroendocrinology, and disorders. In: Kronenberg HM, Melmed S, Polonsky KS and Larsen PR, editors. Williams Textbook of Endocrinology (11th Edition). Philadelphia, USA: Saunders Elsevier, 2008; p. 1066.

[62] Sanders JE. Growth and development after hematopoietic cell transplant in children. Bone Marrow Transplant. 2008;41:223–227. DOI: 10.1038/sj.bmt.1705875

[63] Giorgiani G, Bozzola M, Locatelli F, Picco P, Zecca M, Cisternino M, Dallorso S, Bonetti F, Dini G, Borrone C, Regazzi MB, De Stefano P, Severi F. Role of busulfan and total body irradiation on growth of prepubertal children receiving bone marrow transplantation and results of treatment with recombinant human growth hormone. Blood. 1995;86:825–831.

[64] Isfan F, Kanold J, Merlin E, Contet A, Sirvent N, Rochette E, Poiree M, Terral D, Carla-Malpuech H, Reynaud R, Pereira B, Chastagner P, Simeoni MC, Auquier P, Michel G, Deméocq F. Growth hormone treatment impact on growth rate and final height of patients who received HSCT with TBI or/and cranial irradiation in childhood: a report from the French Leukaemia Long-Term Follow-Up Study (LEA). Bone Marrow Transplant. 2012;47:684–693. DOI: 10.1038/bmt.2011.139

[65] Bell J, Parker KL, Swinford RD, Hoffman AR, Maneatis T, Lippe B. Long-term safety of recombinant human growth hormone in children. J Clin Endocrinol Metab. 2010;95:167–177. DOI: 10.1210/jc.2009-0178

[66] Meazza C, Pagani S, Pietra B, Tinelli C, Calcaterra V, Bozzola E, Bozzola M. Different long-term response to growth hormone therapy in small- versus appropriate-for-gestational-age children with growth hormone deficiency. Horm Res Paediatr. 2013;79:214–219. DOI: 10.1159/000350239

[67] Kriström B, Dahlgren J, Niklasson A, Nierop AF, Albertsson-Wikland K. The first-year growth response to growth hormone treatment predicts the long-term prepubertal growth response in children. BMC Med Inform Decis Mak. 2009;9:1. DOI: 10.1186/1472-6947-9-1

[68] Ranke MB, Lindberg A, Chatelain P, Wilton P, Cutfield W, Albertsson-Wikland K, Price DA. Derivation and validation of a mathematical model for predicting the response to exogenous recombinant human growth hormone (GH) in prepubertal children with idiopathic GH deficiency. KIGS International Board. Kabi Pharmacia International Growth Study. J Clin Endocrinol Metab. 1999;84:1174–1183.

[69] Cuttler L, Silvers JB, Singh J, Tsai AC, Radcliffe D. Physician decisions to discontinue long-term medications using a two-stage framework: the case of growth hormone therapy. Med Care. 2005;43:1185–1193.

[70] Hardin DS, Kemp SF, Allen DB. Twenty years of recombinant human growth hormone in children: relevance to pediatric care providers. Clin Pediatr (Phila). 2007;46:279–286. DOI: 10.1177/0009922806293924

[71] Jorge AA, Marchisotti FG, Montenegro LR, Carvalho LR, Mendonca BB, Arnhold IJ. Growth hormone (GH) pharmacogenetics: influence of GH receptor exon 3 retention or deletion on first-year growth response and final height in patients with severe GH deficiency. J Clin Endocrinol Metab. 2006;91:1076–1080. DOI: http://dx.doi.org/10.1210/jc.2005-2005

[72] Dos Santos C, Essioux L, Teinturier C, Tauber M, Goffin V, Bougnères P. A common polymorphism of the growth hormone receptor is associated with increased responsiveness to growth hormone. Nat Genet. 2004;36:720–724. DOI: 10.1038/ng1379

[73] Räz B, Janner M, Petkovic V, Lochmatter D, Eblé A, Dattani MT, Hindmarsh PC, Flück CE, Mullis PE. Influence of growth hormone (GH) receptor deletion of exon 3 and full-length isoforms on GH response and final height in patients with severe GH deficiency. J Clin Endocrinol Metab. 2008;93:974–980. DOI: http://dx.doi.org/10.1210/jc.2007-1382#sthash.t73ih4HP.dpuf

[74] Pilotta A, Mella P, Filisetti M, Felappi B, Prandi E, Parrinello G, Notarangelo LD, Buzi F. Common polymorphisms of the growth hormone (GH) receptor do not correlate with the growth response to exogenous recombinant human GH in GH-deficient children. J Clin Endocrinol Metab. 2006;91:1178–1180. DOI: http://dx.doi.org/10.1210/jc.2005-1308#sthash.roEyDGce.dpuf

[75] Blum WF, Machinis K, Shavrikova EP, Keller A, Stobbe H, Pfaeffle RW, Amselem S. The growth response to growth hormone (GH) treatment in children with isolated GH deficiency is independent of the presence of the exon 3-minus isoform of the GH receptor. J Clin Endocrinol Metab. 2006;91:4171–4174. DOI: http://dx.doi.org/10.1210/jc.2006-0063

[76] de Graaff LC, Meyer S, Els C, Hokken-Koelega AC. GH receptor d3 polymorphism in Dutch patients with MPHD and IGHD born small or appropriate for gestational age. Clin Endocrinol (Oxf). 2008;68:930–934. DOI:10.1111/j.1365-2265.2007.03140.x

[77] Marchisotti FG, Jorge AA, Montenegro LR, Berger K, de Carvalho LR, Mendonca BB, Arnhold IJ. Comparison between weight-based and IGF1-based growth hormone (GH) dosing in the treatment of children with GH deficiency and influence of exon 3 deleted GH receptor variant. Growth Horm IGF Res. 2009;19:179–186. DOI:10.1016/j.ghir.2008.10.001

[78] Moyes VJ, Walker DM, Owusu-Antwi S, Maher KT, Metherell L, Akker SA, Monson JP, Clark AJ, Drake WM. d3-GHR genotype does not explain heterogeneity in GH responsiveness in hypopituitary adults. Clin Endocrinol (Oxf). 2010;72:807–813. DOI: 10.1111/j.1365-2265.2009.03768.x

[79] Valsesia A, Chatelain P, Stevens A, Peterkova VA, Belgorosky A, Maghnie M, Antoniazzi F, Koledova E, Wojcik J, Farmer P, Destenaves B, Clayton P; PREDICT Investigator group. GH deficiency status combined with GH receptor polymorphism affects response to GH in children. Eur J Endocrinol. 2015;173:777–789. DOI: 10.1530/EJE-15-0474

[80] Wan L, Chen WC, Tsai Y, Kao YT, Hsieh YY, Lee CC, Tsai CH, Chen CP, Tsai FJ. Growth hormone (GH) receptor C.1319 G>T polymorphism, but not exon 3 retention or deletion is associated with better first-year growth response to GH therapy in patients with GH deficiency. Pediatr Res. 2007;62:735–740. DOI: 10.1203/01.pdr.0000290803.86985.61

[81] Buzi F, Mella P, Pilotta A, Prandi E, Lanfranchi F, Carapella T. Growth hormone receptor polymorphisms. In: Lorini R, Maghnie M, D'Annunzio G, Loche S and Savage MO, editors. Congenital Endocrinopathies. New Insights into Endocrine Diseases and Diabetes. Endocrine Development. Basel, Switzerland: Karger, 2007; 11: p 28–35. DOI: 10.1159/000111055

[82] Braz AF, Costalonga EF, Trarbach EB, Scalco RC, Malaquias AC, Guerra-Junior G, Antonini SR, Mendonca BB, Arnhold IJ, Jorge AA. Genetic predictors of long-term response to growth hormone (GH) therapy in children with GH deficiency and Turner syndrome: the influence of a SOCS2 polymorphism. J Clin Endocrinol Metab. 2014;99:E1808–E1813. DOI: 10.1210/jc.2014-1744

[83] Haverkamp F, Johansson L, Dumas H, Langham S, Tauber M, Veimo D, Chiarelli F. Observations of nonadherence to recombinant human growth hormone therapy in clinical practice. Clin Ther. 2008;30:307–316. DOI: 10.1016/j.clinthera.2008.02.017

[84] Fisher BG, Acerini CL. Understanding the growth hormone therapy adherence paradigm: a systematic review. Horm Res Paediatr. 2013;79:189–196. DOI: 10.1159/000350251

[85] Hindmarsh PC, Brook CG. Compliance with growth hormone treatment–is it a problem? Horm Res. 1999;51:104–108. DOI: 10.1159/000053170

[86] Stephenson BJ, Rowe BH, Haynes RB, Macharia WM, Leon G. The rational clinical examination. Is this patient taking the treatment as prescribed? JAMA. 1993;269:2779–2781. DOI: 10.1001/jama.1993.03500210079036

[87] Ingersoll KS, Cohen J. The impact of medication regimen factors on adherence to chronic treatment: a review of literature. J Behav Med. 2008;31:213–224. DOI: 10.1007/s10865-007-9147-y

[88] Cromer BA, Tarnowski KJ. Noncompliance in adolescents: a review. J Dev Behav Pediatr. 1989;10:207–215.

[89] Bozzola M, Pagani S, Iughetti L, Maffeis C, Bozzola E, Meazza C. Adherence to growth hormone therapy: a practical approach. Horm Res Paediatr. 2014;81:331–335. DOI: 10.1159/000357975

[90] Fillion M, Deal C, Van Vliet G. Retrospective study of the potential benefits and adverse events during growth hormone treatment in children with Prader-Willi syndrome. J Pediatr. 2009;154:230–233. DOI: 10.1016/j.jpeds.2008.07.058

[91] Meazza C, Schaab M, Pagani S, Calcaterra V, Bozzola E, Kratzsch J, Bozzola M. Development of antibodies against growth hormone (GH) during rhGH therapy in a girl with

idiopathic GH deficiency: a case report. J Pediatr Endocrinol Metab. 2013;26:785–788. DOI: 10.1515/jpem-2013-0064

[92] Swerdlow AJ, Cooke R, Albertsson-Wikland K, Borgström B, Butler G, Cianfarani S, Clayton P, Coste J, Deodati A, Ecosse E, Gausche R, Giacomozzi C, Kiess W, Hokken-Koelega AC, Kuehni CE, Landier F, Maes M, Mullis PE, Pfaffle R, Sävendahl L, Sommer G, Thomas M, Tollerfield S, Zandwijken GR, Carel JC. Description of the SAGhE Cohort: a large European study of mortality and cancer incidence risks after childhood treatment with recombinant growth hormone. Horm Res Paediatr. 2015;84:172–183. DOI: 10.1159/000435856

[93] Carel JC, Ecosse E, Landier F, Meguellati-Hakkas D, Kaguelidou F, Rey G, Coste J. Long-term mortality after recombinant growth hormone treatment for isolated growth hormone deficiency or childhood short stature: preliminary report of the French SAGhE study. J Clin Endocrinol Metab. 2012;97:416–425. DOI: 10.1210/jc.2011-1995

[94] Sävendahl L, Maes M, Albertsson-Wikland K, Borgström B, Carel JC, Henrard S, Speybroeck N, Thomas M, Zandwijken G, Hokken-Koelega A. Long-term mortality and causes of death in isolated GHD, ISS, and SGA patients treated with recombinant growth hormone during childhood in Belgium, The Netherlands, and Sweden: preliminary report of 3 countries participating in the EU SAGhE study. J Clin Endocrinol Metab. 2012;97:E213–E217. DOI: 10.1210/jc.2011-2882

[95] Mo D, Hardin DS, Erfurth EM, Melmed S. Adult mortality or morbidity is not increased in childhood-onset growth hormone deficient patients who received pediatric GH treatment: an analysis of the Hypopituitary Control and Complications Study (HypoCCS). Pituitary. 2014;17:477–485. DOI: 10.1007/s11102-013-0529-6

[96] Ho KK, 2007 GH Deficiency Consensus Workshop Participants. Consensus guidelines for the diagnosis and treatment of adults with GH deficiency II: a statement of the GH Research Society in association with the European Society for Paediatric Endocrinology, Lawson Wilkins Society, European Society of Endocrinology, Japan Endocrine Society, and Endocrine Society of Australia. Eur J Endocrinol. 2007;157:695–700. DOI: 10.1530/EJE-07-0631

[97] Molitch ME, Clemmons DR, Malozowski S, Merriam GR, Vance ML, Endocrine Society. Evaluation and treatment of adult growth hormone deficiency: an Endocrine Society clinical practice guideline. J Clin Endocrinol Metab. 2011;96:1587–1609. DOI: 10.1210/jc.2011-0179

[98] Attanasio AF, Howell S, Bates PC, Blum WF, Frewer P, Quigley C, Shalet SM. Confirmation of severe GH deficiency after final height in patients diagnosed as GH deficient during childhood. Clin Endocrinol. 2002;56:503–507. DOI: 10.1046/j.1365-2265.2002.01515.x

[99] Smyczyńska J, Stawerska R, Lewiński A, Hilczer M. Incidence and predictors of persistent growth hormone deficiency (GHD) in patients with isolated, childhood-onset GHD. Endokrynol Pol. 2014;65:334–341. DOI: 10.5603/EP.2014.0046

[100] Deillon E, Hauschild M, Faouzi M, Stoppa-Vaucher S, Elowe-Gruau E, Dwyer A, Theintz GE, Dubuis JM, Mullis PE, Pitteloud N, Phan-Hug F. Natural history of growth hormone deficiency in a pediatric cohort. Horm Res Paediatr. 2015;83:252–261. DOI: 10.1159/000369392

[101] Bizzarri C, Pedicelli S, Boscherini B, Bedogni G, Cappa M, Cianfarani S. Early retesting by GHRH+arginine test shows normal GH response in most children with idiopathic GH deficiency. J Endocrinol Invest. 2015;38:429–436. DOI: 10.1007/s40618-014-0205-3

[102] Maghnie M, Aimaretti G, Bellone S, Bona G, Bellone J, Baldelli R, de Sanctis C, Gargantini L, Gastaldi R, Ghizzoni L, Secco A, Tinelli C, Ghigo E. Diagnosis of GH deficiency in the transition period: accuracy of insulin tolerance test and insulin-like growth factor-I measurement. Eur J Endocrinol. 2005;152:589–196. DOI: 10.1530/eje. 1.01873

[103] Secco A, di Iorgi N, Napoli F, Calandra E, Calcagno A, Ghezzi M, Frassinetti C, Fratangeli N, Parodi S, Benassai M, Leitner Y, Gastaldi R, Lorini R, Maghnie M, Radetti G. Reassessment of the growth hormone status in young adults with childhood-onset growth hormone deficiency: reappraisal of insulin tolerance testing. J Clin Endocrinol Metab. 2009;94:4195–4204. DOI: 10.1210/jc.2009-0602

[104] Chesover AD, Dattani MT. Evaluation of Growth Hormone Stimulation Testing in Children. Clin Endocrinol (Oxf). 2016;84:708–714. DOI: 10.1111/cen.13035.

[105] Cappa M, Caruso M, Saggese G, Salerno MC, Tonini G. GH therapy in transition age: state of the art and future perspectives. Minerva Endocrinol. 2015;40:23–35.

[106] Mullis PE. Genetics of GHRH, GHRH-receptor, GH and GH-receptor: its impact on pharmacogenetics. Best Pract Res Clin Endocrinol Metab. 2011;25:25–41. DOI: 10.1016/ j.beem.2010.06.006

[107] Alatzoglou KS, Webb EA, Le Tissier P, Dattani MT. Isolated growth hormone deficiency (GHD) in childhood and adolescence: recent advances. Endocr Rev. 2014;35:376–432. DOI: 10.1210/er.2013-1067

[108] Inoue H, Kangawa N, Kinouchi A, Sakamoto Y, Kimura C, Horikawa R, Shigematsu Y, Itakura M, Ogata T, Fujieda K; Japan Growth Genome Consortium. Identification and functional analysis of novel human growth hormone secretagogue receptor (GHSR) gene mutations in Japanese subjects with short stature. J Clin Endocrinol Metab. 2011;96:E373–E378. DOI: 10.1210/jc.2010-1570

[109] Alatzoglou KS, Dattani MT. Genetic forms of hypopituitarism and their manifestation in the neonatal period. Early Hum Dev. 2009;85:705–712. DOI: 10.1016/j.earlhumdev. 2009.08.057

[110] Pfäffle R, Klammt J. Pituitary transcription factors in the aetiology of combined pituitary hormone deficiency. Best Pract Res Clin Endocrinol Metab. 2011;25:43–60. DOI: 10.1016/j.beem.2010.10.014

[111] Correa FA, Trarbach EB, Tusset C, Latronico AC, Montenegro LR, Carvalho LR, Franca MM, Otto AP, Costalonga EF, Brito VN, Abreu AP, Nishi MY, Jorge AA, Arnhold IJ, Sidis Y, Pitteloud N, Mendonca BB. FGFR1 and PROKR2 rare variants found in patients with combined pituitary hormone deficiencies. Endocr Connect. 2015;4:100–107. DOI: 10.1530/EC-15-0015

Chapter 3

Genetic Determinants of Short Stature

Diana Miclea

Additional information is available at the end of the chapter

http://dx.doi.org/10.5772/64561

Abstract

Growth in height is a multifactorial process in which 80–90% of the contributing factors are genetic. The genes that determine the appropriate morphology and function of the skeletal and endocrinal system are the most being involved. Short stature is a clinical sign noted in conditions that intrinsically affect the growth plate, such as skeletal dysplasia, or in genetic syndromes such as Turner's, Silver-Russell, Noonan's, Cornelia de Lange's, Rubinstein-Taybi and Prader-Willi syndrome. Also, some endocrine diseases or chronic disorders can lead to change growth in the plate physiology, leading to short stature; the endocrine disorders are often genetically determined. Another category is idiopathic short stature, which is the most important in terms of frequency, and even though in this case, the aetiology is not proven; it seems that the genetic factors have the main role. In this chapter, the genetic syndromes with primary effect on growth are presented and the principal aim is to highlight the main clinical signs associated with short stature, which can lead to an easier clinical diagnosis of a genetic disease that mainly influence growth, thus facilitating the selection of the genetic test needed for the etiologic diagnosis in short stature.

Keywords: short stature, skeletal dysplasia, genetic syndromes, genetic testing

1. Introduction

Growth is defined as elongation and maturation of the bones and is a multifactorial process; more than 80% of growth is contributed by coordination of genetic factors [1]. Genetic influence is argued by the height difference observed in different ethnic populations or in different families. An argument for the role of environmental factors is done by the secular trend of growth observed in the last 150 years and is usually correlated with a better socio-economic status [2].

In order to understand the effect of genes on processes of growth, it is important to know about 'major genes' and 'minor genes' [3]. 'The major genes' have a critical role on growth, and single mutations in them usually results in growth pathology (monogenic disorders) [3]. Mutations of 'the minor genes' only provide a susceptibility for growth abnormalities (multifactorial disorders) [3] whose effect being validated as a disease when multiple genetic and environmental factors act together.

A mutation of a 'major gene' (monogenic disease) is usually considered, when the short stature is severe, under -3DS or when the short stature is associated with malformative syndrome or/and dysmorphic features or/and intellectual disability or there is an evidence for skeletal dysplasia or microcephaly or small for gestational age (SGA) without catch-up growth or severe growth hormone (GH) deficiency or multiple pituitary hormones deficits [4]. The mutations of 'minor genes' are usually conducted to a growth phenotype that is only slightly affected (familial or constitutional short stature), this effect being multifactorial determined.

Concerning 'the minor genes', the genome-wide association studies (GWAS) demonstrated that there are more than 180 genetic variants correlated with growth, on autosomes, with independent, additional effect of 0.2–0.6 cm for every allele [5, 6]. Also, it was also observed that there are two types of genes: 'height genes', having the main role in adult height, and 'tempo genes' , important for the starting moment of the different processes of growth [6, 7]. Genetic factors act mainly through skeletal and endocrine systems.

Short stature represents a height under -2DS for the average of general population of the same age, sex and ethnicity. A useful classification of the aetiology in short stature divides it into primary, secondary and idiopathic short statures.

Primary short stature includes intrinsic conditions of the growth plate (15–20% of cases) [8], such as skeletal dysplasia, genetic syndromes (Turner, Down, DiGeorge, Silver-Russell, Noonan, Cornelia de Lange, Rubenstein-Taybi, Prader-Willi and neurofibromatosis type I) and SGA with failure of catch-up growth.

Secondary short stature refers to conditions that change growth plate physiology (30–35% of cases) [8], such as endocrine disorders, chronic disorders in different organ and systems, insufficient nutrient intake (malnutrition) and metabolic or psychosocial disorders.

Idiopathic short stature (50% of cases) [8] includes familial short stature, non-familial short stature and constitutional growth and puberty delay.

In every category, the genetic aetiology is obvious for a great number of disorders, especially in primary short stature and endocrine disorders. Even in idiopathic short stature, it was observed that in more than 20% of cases, there is a subtle skeletal dysplasia that is also genetically determined [9], 4% of them were demonstrated to have short stature homeobox (SHOX) gene deletion [10]. Also in familial idiopathic short stature, the genetic background is evident.

In this chapter, the disorders included in the category primary short stature, where genetic factors have a clearer contribution and where usually one major gene is implicated in the processes of abnormal growth, will be mainly presented. In the genetic evaluation of a child with short stature, 'the major genes' are usually searched, the others, such as 'minor genes', give only a predisposition and are considered only after the exclusion of the major factors. An adequate genetic evaluation usually facilitates decisions about therapeutic intervention and gives clues about the prognosis.

2. Genetic disorders with primary effect on growth

2.1. Skeletal dysplasia

The specific clinical trait of the skeletal dysplasia is a disproportionate short stature, with associated signs such as shorter and bowed long bones, shorter ribs, polydactyly, impaired bone density and bone modelling, disorganized development of growth cartilage and ossification defects. Growth retardation is seen in some skeletal dysplasia beginning with intrauterine life or, for others, has a post-natal onset in the first year of life or even later in some cases. The diagnosis is usually established by clinical and radiological signs. Molecular analysis for confirmation is required particularly in the situation of genetic counselling in order to evaluate a future pregnancy by pre-natal diagnosis. Otherwise, sometimes a skeletal dysplasia can be diagnosed even for a patient with isolated short stature, apparently proportionate, whom only a radiological assessment may show the signs of dysplasia [9].

Skeletal dysplasia is a group of disorders, and is very heterogeneous; clinically and molecularly, more than 400 syndromes have been described, the more recent classification dividing them into 40 principal groups [11]. Skeletal dysplasia without identified molecular bases is also identified. In the following section, the most common and molecularly well-characterized skeletal dysplasia are presented.

2.1.1. The FGFR3-related chondrodysplasias

The *FGFR* gene (4p16.3) encodes for *fibroblast growth factor receptor 3* that has a main effect in the regulation of chondrocyte proliferation, differentiation and apoptosis [12, 13]. *FGFR3* regulates osteogenesis and post-natal bone mineralization by osteoblasts, the main role being in endochondral ossification [12, 13]. It has an extracellular region with three immunoglobulin-like domains, a transmembrane domain and an intracellular region with tyrosine kinase domains. Mutations in *FGFR3* gene lead to several syndromes with a phenotype more or less severe according to the affected region of the receptor, such as achondroplasia, hypochondroplasia, SADDAN syndrome (Severe Achondroplasia with Developmental Delay and Acanthosis Nigricans) and thanatophoric dysplasia. The *FGFR3* mutations responsible for these syndromes are mutations with gain of function, inducing an activation of the receptor.

2.1.1.1. Achondroplasia

It is the most known form of disproportionate short stature and has a frequency of 1:25,000 births. In achondroplasia, *FGFR3* gene mutations affect the transmembrane region of the receptor [14]. Note that 98% of cases show G1138A mutation, an additional 1% of cases presenting the G1138C mutation [15, 16]. Achondroplasia is an autosomal dominant disorder with complete penetrance. About 80% of cases occur as a result of *de novo* mutations, often produced in paternal gametes, usually in case of an advanced paternal age at procreation [17]. These mutations are activating ones and affect mainly the endochondral ossification, with impact on hypertrophic cellular compartment, chondrocyte proliferation in growth cartilages and cartilage formation [12, 13].

Disproportionate short stature is a characteristic of the disease, adult height usually not exceeding 125–130 cm. The clinical picture is represented by the specific skeletal features: short rhizomelic limbs, relative macrocephaly, frontal bossing with mid-face hypoplasia, trident hands and hyperlordosis. The patients had associated with hypotonia (at young age) and obesity (often in adults).

2.1.1.2. Hypochondroplasia

Hypochondroplasia is a pathology often produced by *FGFR3* mutations in the extracellular or intracellular region in the proximal tyrosine kinase domain [16]. In 70% of cases, *FGFR3* mutations are described [18]. Some authors have noticed, in some cases, the association of hypochondroplasia with *IGF1* mutations [19]. There are some cases for which genetic determinant is not yet identified. Thus, unlike the achondroplasia, the hypochondroplasia is characterised by genetic heterogeneity.

The clinical picture is that of a mild achondroplasia and is represented by disproportionate short stature with short limbs but without an obvious rhizomelia, brachydactyly affected spine by narrowing the interpediculate distance at the lumbar level [20]. Final height is not as severely affected as in achondroplasia and is usually in the range 130–165 cm.

2.1.1.3. SADDAN syndrome

SADDAN syndrome is a severe form of achondroplasia associated with developmental delay and *acanthosis nigricans,* the name of syndrome being an acronym of the main clinical signs. In these disorders, a *FGFR3* missense mutation Lys650Met was described, located at the distal tyrosine kinase domain [21]. This mutation is located in the same codon as the specific mutations that produce thanatophoric dysplasia.

Patients have bone dysplasia as described in achondroplasia, but more severe are important short stature, micromelia, macrocephaly, frontal bossing, wide anterior fontanelle, mid-face hypoplasia, bowed tibia and narrow thorax [22]. In addition, they also have progressive *acanthosis nigricans,* CNS abnormalities, epilepsy and severe developmental delay [21]. SADDAN syndrome clinically overlaps with thanatophoric dysplasia, but survival in the first one is beyond the neo-natal period, cases with this pathology are even reported in young adulthood.

2.1.1.4. Thanatophoric dysplasia

It is the most common lethal skeletal dysplasia in the neo-natal period. Two subtypes have been described: thanatophoric dysplasia type I, caused by mutations in the extracellular or intracellular region of *FGFR3* gene, and thanatophoric dysplasia type II, which is produced by mutations at the distal tyrosine kinase domain [23, 24]. The most common mutation in type I is R248C, confirmed in about 50% of the patients [24]. In type II, the K650E mutation is the only one reported, which is present in more than 99% of the patients [23, 24].

The two forms of thanatophoric dysplasia were divided according to the clinical picture. In type I, the clinical characteristics are the short and bowed long bones with skull normal appearance [25, 26]. In type II, the traits are represented by the cloverleaf skull with short and straight long bones [25]. Other associated signs, common to the two types are: platyspondyly, narrow and short thorax, ventriculomegaly and polyhydramnios [25].

2.1.2. Disorders produced by abnormalities of collagen and other extracellular structural protein

2.1.2.1. Osteogenesis imperfecta

It occurs in 95% of cases due to *COL1A1* (17q21.33) and *COL1A2* (7q21.3) mutations, genes encoding $\alpha 1$ and $\alpha 2$ polypeptide chains of type I collagen [27]. Type I collagen is the most abundant collagen found in extracellular matrix protein and it is mainly present in cartilage, bone, ligaments, tegument, dentin and sclera [28, 29]. Its role is structural, which interacts with other matrix proteins (proteoglycans or fibronectins) and with the cells by anchoring them into the matrix. A functional role was also described in signalling receptors on surface cells to regulate cell growth, motility and differentiation [28–30].

The mutations of the chains of type I collagen lead to quantitative or qualitative impairment and the clinical picture will be represented by the signs of the organs more abundant in type I collagen: bones, articulations, dentin and sclera. These signs are multiple fractures arisen usually after minor traumatisms, bone deformities, short stature, osteoporosis, joint hyper-laxity, *dentinogenesis imperfecta*, blues sclera, deafness and wormian bones. The skeletal impairment is secondary to osseous fragility and osteopenia. Short stature is observed usually secondary to the pathologic bone and its deformities. There are several clinical forms of osteogenesis imperfecta, with different degree of severity. In 1979, Sillence and colleagues described the four classical types of osteogenesis [31]. The actual classification includes fifteen types, the first four being the known ones, produced by type I collagen mutations, the others being the result of different gene mutations. Type I is a mild non-deforming form of osteogenesis imperfecta, with a blue sclera and a little or absent effect on growth Type II is the most severe form, lethal in the peri-natal period. The clinical picture is represented by an important osteopenia that leads to multiple fractures, secondary deformities and very short length from the intrauterine period. Type III has also a severe phenotype, but less than the type II, represented by very short stature, deformities, *dentinogenesis imperfecta* and blue sclera. Type IV has an intermediate severity with a mild short stature, moderate deformities after recurrent fractures, *dentinogenesis imperfecta* and normal sclera. If the chains of type I collagen are affected, the transmission is autosomal dominant. In 5% of cases, osteogenesis imperfecta is secondary to mutations of different genes, such as *SERPINF1* (17p13.3), *LEPRE1* (1p34.1), *CRTAP* (3p22), *PPIB* (15q21-q22), *SERPINH1* (11q13.5), *FKBP10* (17q21.2), *SP7* (12q13.13), *BMP1* (8p21.3),

TMEM38B (9q31.2) and WNT1 (12q13.12); these disorders having an autosomal recessive transmission, usually with a severe clinical phenotype [27].

2.1.2.2. Skeletal dysplasia in type II collagen abnormalities

Type II collagen is mostly found in cartilage, intervertebral disc and eye, and various mutations lead to a group of diseases that have in common the abnormalities of epiphysis, spine and eyes, which can easily be recognized by the signs in these structures [32]. The disorders of this group of pathologies are specifically produced by different mutations of the same gene *COL2A1* (12q13.11) that encodes for $\alpha 1$ chain of type II collagen [32]. The majority of *COL2A1* mutations were observed in the triple-helical region of alpha 1 chain [33]. These disorders have an autosomal dominant transmission. However, they are often produced by *de novo* mutations and show a great variability of clinical expression.

2.1.2.2.1. Achondrogenesis

Achondrogenesis is one of the most severe skeletal dysplasia, with an important lethality, in foetal life or in the neo-natal period. There are two forms that differ by the type of transmission (type I, recessive, and type II, dominant) and by the length and structure of long bones. The clinical picture is characterized by very small length, extreme micromelia, very short trunk, vertebral, skull and pelvis ossification defects, cupping metaphysis, cystic hygroma and polyhydramnios [34]. Type II is secondary to neo-mutations in type II collagen and is less severe than achondrogenesis type I that is produced by *TRIP11* or *DTDST* mutations. Achondrogenesis type II is the most severe pathology of type II collagen group of disorders. Hypochondrogenesis represents a mild form of achondrogenesis type II and is also produced by mutations in type II collagen [35].

2.1.2.2.2. Spondyloepiphyseal dysplasia congenita

It is characterized by poor somatic growth since intrauterine life. An important associated sign is vertebral dysplasia, usually seen as platyspondyly. Other abnormalities often seen in this disorder are cleft palate, ophthalmologic abnormalities (myopia, nystagmus, cataracts and retinal detachment) and deafness. Short stature is also an important sign in the post-natal period, the height not exceeding 130 cm, other signs of skeletal dysplasia being deformation of femoral head with a secondary *coxa vara*, scoliosis and impaired cervical spine [36]. There is a significant clinical variability, the clinical spectrum including various forms of severity. The responsible mutations that occur are missense mutations that substitute bulky amino acids for glycine residues in the triple-helical region of $\alpha 1$ chain of type II collagen [33].

2.1.2.2.3. Kniest dysplasia

Kniest dysplasia is characterized by extreme short stature, prominent joints, especially in knee, and mid-face hypoplasia. It is also associated with myopia, deafness or cleft palate. At vertebral region, platyspondyly can be seen with vertical clefts, kyphoscoliosis or hyperlordosis [37]. Epiphysis is generally large, especially in the knee. The femoral head is often absent due to a developmental defect of the femoral epiphysis and the iliac bones are characteristically shaped [37]. In Kniest dysplasia, the α1 chain of type II collagen is modified by exon skipping due to splice-site mutations in the region encoding the triple-helical region [33].

2.1.2.2.4. Stickler dysplasia type I

Stickler dysplasia is characterized by genetic heterogeneity, the mutations in type II collagen or type XI collagen being responsible for this pathology. The abnormalities of type II collagen lead to Stickler dysplasia type I. The haploinsufficiency of truncation mutations that occur in the triple-helical region of α1 chain of type II collagen is responsible for the phenotype [33]. This syndrome also presents a clinical variability. The main clinical signs are represented by skeletal and ophthalmologic disorders (high myopia and retinal detachment), auditory abnormalities (deafness) and craniofacial dysmorphia (mid-face hypoplasia, micrognathia, midline cleft of the face and Pierre Robin sequence) [38, 39]. The patients usually present a short stature associated with a moderate spondyloepiphyseal dysplasia [39]. Radiologic signs are often minor, such as discreet flattening and irregularities at the epiphyseal region or a minimum platyspondyly, especially in the dorsal region. Patients associate widening joints, especially in the knee, and osteoarthritis with early onset [39].

2.1.2.3. Skeletal dysplasia in type IX collagen, cartilage oligomeric matrix protein (COMP) and matrilin 3 (MATN3) abnormalities

Type IX collagen, *cartilage oligomeric matrix protein* and *matrilin 3* are components of the cartilage extracellular matrix that strongly interacts to maintain cartilage assembly and integrity [40, 41]. A mutation of one of these components modifies the secretion of the others and the common pathology produced for each gene mutation is multiple epiphyseal dysplasia (MED) [41]. The pathogenesis is represented by the impairment of endochondral ossification due to cartilage abnormalities.

There are six types of MED produced by mutations of *COMP* (19p13.1) (MED type I), *COL9A2* (1p32.2–33) (MED type II), *COL9A3* (20q13.3) (MED type III), *DTDST* (5q32–33) (MED type IV), *MATN3* (2p23–24) (MED type V) and *COL9A1* (6q13) (MED type VI) [11]. With the exception of MED type IV, all these disorders are transmitted in autosomal dominant manner. All these types share a common clinical picture; some particularities being observed in each type. The most specific signs of these disorders are short stature and precocious osteoarthritis. Characteristically, the patients present pain and precocious fatigability when a physical activity is initiated. The phenotypic signs are observed only post-natally, after an apparently normal initial development. Even if the skeletal impairment is generalized, the bones of inferior limbs are more frequently involved, being often observed an angular deformation at this level, such as *coxa vara, genu varum, genu valgum* and *valgum* deformities at the distal tibia.

The mutations of α1, α2 or α3 chain of type IX collagen (*COL9A1, COL9A2, COL9A3*) are associated with a preponderant impairment of the knee [42].

In *COMP* mutations, the impairment of proximal femur and acetabulum is particularly observed [43].

In *MATN3* mutations, the clinical picture is similar with that observed in *COMP* mutations, but less severe [44].

2.1.2.4. Skeletal dysplasia in type X collagen abnormalities

Type X collagen also has an important role in endochondral ossification, influencing the compartmentations of different matrix components and also the regulation of the mineralization [45].

2.1.2.4.1. Metaphyseal chondrodysplasia, Schmid type

It is produced by mutations of $\alpha 1$ chain of type X of collagen gene (*COL1A10*) (6q21–22.3), and the transmission of the disorder is autosomal dominant. It is characterized by moderately short stature with post-natal onset, the size at birth being within normal limits. Radiography showed irregularities in the metaphysis of long bones. The consequence of *COL10A1* mutations is the bowing and the shortening of the long bones, *coxa vara* being usually observed. Often, the patients may develop the spine impairment, such as mild platyspondyly or other abnormalities of the vertebral body.

2.1.2.5. Skeletal dysplasia in type XI collagen abnormalities

Type XI collagen has an important interaction with type II collagen, helping in maintaining the spacing and the architecture of the type II collagen. Two polypeptide chains, $\alpha 1$ and $\alpha 2$, contribute to the formation of type XI collagen; the genes that encode these chains being *COL11A1* (1p21) and *COL11A2* (6p21.3). The mutations in these genes lead to a clinical phenotype of skeletal dysplasia overlapping with that produced by type II collagen abnormalities.

2.1.2.5.1. Stickler dysplasia type II

It is the consequence of *COL11A1* mutations. These mutations lead to a clinical picture similar to that described in Stickler syndrome type I (see Section 2.1.2.2.4), the main clinical signs being the consequence of skeletal, ophthalmologic and auditory impairments. However, the clinical severity is higher in terms of ophthalmologic (severe myopia, bilateral retinal detachment) and auditory (deafness) phenotypes [46]. The craniofacial dysmorphic features that are specific for Stickler syndrome type I or II are as follows: mid-facial hypoplasia, midline clefting and retromicrognatia (Pierre Robin syndrome). The short stature is also seen associated with hip abnormalities, such as slipped capital femoral epiphysis and mild thoracolumbar spinal abnormalities that often lead to scoliosis [47, 48]. The disease has an autosomal dominant transmission.

2.1.2.5.2. Otospondylomegaepiphyseal dysplasia (OSMED syndrome)

This dysplasia is the consequence of *COL11A2* mutations and is also called non-ocular Stickler dysplasia. The disease has an autosomal recessive transmission. Skeletal similarities with Kniest dysplasia is noticed, but without ophthalmologic involvement. However, the hearing impairment is much more important. Thus, the clinical picture is represented by sensorineural hearing loss, disproportionate short stature with micromelia, enlarged epiphyses and spine abnormalities, and dysmorphic facial features [49].

2.1.2.6. Sulfation disorders group

In this group of disorders, the main gene mutated is *DTDST* (5q32–33) that encodes for sulphate transporter SLC26A2 that influences the sulfation of proteoglycans in cartilage matrix [50]. The pathologies of this group are autosomal recessives, in contrast to the previously presented anomalies that are characterized by autosomal dominant inheritance. The disorders produced by *DTDST* mutations are diastrophic dysplasia, achondrogenesis type IB, atelosteogenesis type II and MED type IV [11].

2.1.2.6.1. Diastrophic dysplasia

It is characterized by disproportionate growth retardation with micromelia, debuted in prenatal period [51]. Progressively, after birth, multiple joint contractures occur, especially in the shoulders, elbows, hip and interphalangeal joints [52]. At birth, the congenital club foot, the hypoplasia of the first metacarpal, thumb subluxation or cervical subluxation is also noted. Long bones are short and large [52]. There is a progressive scoliosis. Other specific features are the cysts observed at the ear pavilion [52]. Radiographic findings are metaphyseal widening and epiphyseal dysplasia.

2.1.2.7. Skeletal dysplasia in perlecan disorders

The perlecan is a heparan sulphate proteoglycan that acts as a co-receptor for *FGF2*, thus having a role in intercellular adhesion and in promoting cells proliferation and angiogenesis. The mutations of gene encoding perlecan (*PLC*, 1q36–34) induce different skeletal disorders transmitted by autosomal recessive mode: dyssegmental dysplasia, Silverman-Handmaker type; dyssegmental dysplasia, Rolland-Desbuquois type; and Schwartz-Jampel syndrome [11].

2.1.2.7.1. Dyssegmental dysplasias

They are represented by two disorders, Silverman-Handmaker and Rolland-Desbuquois, which are the forms of neo-natal short-limbed dwarfism. Both are produced by different mutations of the same gene, *PLC*. The Silverman-Handmaker type is the most severe, being lethal in peri-natal period, compared to Rolland-Desbuquois, which is less severe [53]. The skeletal abnormalities are represented by vertebral segmentation associated with long bones impairments that are shorter, larger and bowed [54]. The vertebral segmentation is observed as marked differences in size and shape of vertebral bodies. A reduced joint mobility is often associated. A cleft palate as well as the encephalocele was described.

2.1.2.7.2. Schwartz-Jampel syndrome

It is characterized by short stature, myotonic myopathy, joint contractures, *pectus carinatum*, kyphosis, *coxa valga*, myopia and blepharophimosis [55, 56]. Radiological abnormalities include platyspondyly, short long bones with metaphyseal widening, wide epiphysis of the distal femur and tibia, and fragmented capital femoral epiphysis.

2.1.2.8. Skeletal dysplasia in aggrecan disorders

The aggrecan, also known as cartilage-specific proteoglycan core protein (CSPCP), is a chondroitin sulphate proteoglycan, the most abundant structural component in the cartilage. It leads to a normal chondroskeletal morphogenesis and it also provides a hydrated gel structure in articular cartilage that is important for its resistance [57]. Different mutations of the gene that encodes for aggrecan, *AGC1* (15q26), are responsible for different diseases: spondyloepiphyseal dysplasia, Kimberley type; spondyloepimetaphyseal and metaphyseal dysplasia, aggrecan type; and familial osteochondritis dissecans [11].

2.1.2.8.1. Spondyloepiphyseal dysplasia, Kimberley type

It leads to a proportionate short stature, osteoarthritis with early onset and sometimes to a craniofacial dysmorphia [58]. It is also defined by platyspondyly, vertebral cleft, metaphyseal widening, epiphyseal irregularities and flattening of femoral epiphysis. It is an autosomal dominant pathology.

2.1.2.9. Skeletal disorders in transient receptor potential vanilloid 4 (TRPV4) abnormalities

Transient receptor potential vanilloid 4 (12q24.1) mediates calcium influx, late in osteoclast differentiation, thus influencing bone resorption [59]. *TRPV4* mutations produce not only skeletal pathologies but also non-skeletal (such as spinal muscular atrophy, Charcot-Marie-Tooth disease). The skeletal disorders are transmitted in autosomal dominant mode and include metatropic dysplasia; spondyloepimetaphyseal dysplasia, Maroteaux type; spondylometaphyseal dysplasia, Kozlowski type; brachyolmia; and familial digital arthropathy with brachydactyly [11].

2.1.2.9.1. Metatropic dysplasia

It is a severe form of skeletal dysplasia, often lethal in the neo-natal period, and is characterized by important disproportionate short length in newborn with micromelia, wide metaphyses, platyspondyly, severe kyphoscoliosis, iliac areas in halberd, and limitations and enlargements of the joints [60].

2.1.3. Defects in intracellular structural proteins

2.1.3.1. Filamin group

Although these intracellular structural proteins are expressed in all cells, it has been observed that their mutations often induce a very severe skeletal pathologic phenotype. The filamin A and B are cytoskeleton proteins, their role being structural, in signal transduction, in transport or in intracellular and extracellular communication. Their mutations lead to the absence of some bones or to joint dislocations.

2.1.3.1.1. Filamin A disorders

Mutations of filamin A gene (*FLNA*, Xq28) lead to dominant X-linked disorders. These are: frontometaphyseal dysplasia, otopalatodigital syndromes type I and type II, Melnick-Needles syndrome and terminal osseous dysplasia with pigmentary defects [11].

Frontometaphyseal dysplasia is characterized by skeletal dysplasia, urogenital abnormalities and deafness. Otopalatodigital syndrome type I is characterized by auricular impairment, cleft palate and mild skeletal damage. Type II shows a more pronounced skeletal clinical picture associated with multiple internal malformations (brain, heart and digestive). The Melnick-Needles syndrome is the most severe disorder of filamin A group, being lethal, most often for intrauterine life.

2.1.3.1.2. Filamin B disorders

Mutations of filamin B gene (*FLNB*, 3p14.3) lead to different disorders transmitted in autosomal dominant (the majority) and recessive mode (spondylo-carpal-tarsal dysplasia). These disorders are atelosteogenesis type I, atelosteogenesis type III, Larsen syndrome and spondylocarpotarsal syndrome [11].

Many of these diseases are lethal in the early neo-natal period. In spondylocarpotarsal syndrome, spine fusions were observed. The fusions also implied the carpal and tarsal bones. On the other hand, a hyperlaxity was observed in some joints.

2.1.4. Disorders associated with SHOX gene mutations

Short stature homeobox gene belongs to the paired homeobox family and is localized in the pseudoautosomal region 1 (*PAR1*) of X (Xp22) and Y (Yp11.3) chromosomes. *SHOX* gene is expressed in hypertrophic chondrocytes of the growth plate, having a role in regulating chondrocyte differentiation [61, 62]. The diseases associated with *SHOX* gene abnormalities are Leri-Weill dyschondrosteosis (heterozygous mutations and deletions) and Langer mesomelic dysplasia (homozygous mutations). The skeletal features of Turner syndrome are also a consequence of *SHOX* gene haploinsufficiency. Otherwise, *SHOX* gene mutations were observed at 2–5% of patients with idiopathic isolated short stature [63–65].

SHOX gene is an important determinant of growth, *SHOX* deletions being associated with short stature and *SHOX* duplications with tall stature. *SHOX* gene is expressed in the first and second pharyngeal arches and also in elbow, radius, ulna, and wrist and in the equivalent bones of inferior limbs [66]. Thus, the clinical picture in *SHOX* deficiency is represented by short stature, mesomelia with shortening and bowing of the forearms and tibia, *cubitus valgus*, Madelung deformity of the wrist, brachymetacarpia, brachymetatarsia, high-arched palate, micrognathia and short neck [67]. *SHOX* gene deficiency leads to a marked phenotypic variability, even for the same mutation or in the same family. The clinical picture is more expressed in females and is usually more evident in the beginning of the puberty [68].

2.1.4.1. Leri-Weill dyschondrosteosis

It is the most common form of mesomelic dysplasia and is characterized by disproportionate short stature (145–155 cm) with mesomelia and Madelung deformity [67]. There is an important clinical variability, even in the same family, the females often being more affected. Short stature is observed from the childhood, even from the first year and usually the amplitude of the growth deficiency is correlated with the degree of wrist deformity [67]. The causes of Leri-Weill dyschondrosteosis are heterozygous mutations or deletions of *SHOX* gene.

2.1.4.2. Langer mesomelic dysplasia

It is secondary to homozygous mutations of *SHOX* gene and the clinical picture is represented by severe short stature (-6DS and -7DS) with severe abnormalities of the limbs: hypoplasia and aplasia of the ulna and fibula [67].

2.2. Genetic syndromes with primary effect on growth

2.2.1. Turner syndrome

The Turner syndrome is due to complete or partial loss of one of the two sex chromosomes, homogeneous or in mosaic, in a female patient. Only 50% of the cases present the classical homogeneous monosomy 45,X, the other half having X chromosome mosaicism, X chromosome structural abnormalities (deletions, ring chromosome and isochromosome) or Y chromosome abnormalities (2–5%). The phenotypic features are represented by short stature, dysmorphic syndrome, gonadal dysgenesis and internal malformations. There is a great variability of phenotypic traits, clinical spectrum including complete forms and more often partial forms, represented sometimes only by short stature.

Short stature is the most constant clinical sign, observed in up to 98% of patients [69, 70]. It is secondary to SHOX gene haploinsufficiency. The growth retardation might be seen in about half of patients beginning with pre-natal life [70]. In the others, the short stature will be developed usually after the age of 3–4 years, due to a diminished velocity of growth. The growth worsens progressively until 10 years and the lack of puberty growth spurt will accentuate the deficit. Finally, height will be usually between the interval 122–147 cm [71].

The dysmorphias include triangular face, epicanthus, down-slanted palpebral fissure, macrostomy, high-arched palate, dental abnormalities, micrognathia, low posterior hair insertion line ‘in trident’, *pterygium colli*, large thorax, *cubitus valgus*, short IV and/or V metacarpals, *genu valgum*, extremities lymphedema at birth, multiple pigmented nevi and dysplastic nails [70].

The puberty delay is one of the most common signs being observed in up to 95% of cases [70].

Most patients with Turner syndrome show a normal intellectual development, excepting those presenting ring X chromosome, who often present intellectual disability [72].

Cardiovascular malformations are particularly important in terms of evolution and prognosis, being found in 25–40% of cases [69, 70]. The most specific cardiac abnormalities are bicuspid aortic valve and aortic coarctation. Reno-urinary malformations are observed in 40–60% of the cases, the most representative being horseshoe kidney, polycystic kidney, renal agenesis and duplicated collecting system [71].

Bone abnormalities, affecting more than 60% of patients, have a significant contribution to the external phenotype of the Turner syndrome. Typically, these patients present a lower value for upper segment/lower segment ratio, short neck, large thorax, scoliosis, kyphosis, *cubitus valgus*, Madelung deformity, congenital hip dislocation, *genu valgum*, and short IV and/or V metacarpal and metatarsal [63, 70].

2.2.2. Russell-Silver syndrome

It represents a genetic pathology in which the short stature is the most specific sign. It is very heterogeneous in terms of genetic aetiology and in many cases (about 50%) with typical clinical picture, the aetiology is unknown. Note that 40% of patients present hypomethylation of imprinting centre 1 (IC1) (*H19*, 11p15) [73, 74]. This hypomethylation could occur by epigenetic mechanisms or by duplications of maternal chromosome in 11p15 region. About 10% of patients present maternal uniparental disomy of chromosome 7 [73]. There were reported cases with 17q25 translocations, ring chromosome 2 or other structural abnormalities of 1, 15 or X chromosomes that also had a clinical phenotype of Russell-Silver syndrome [75–77].

The clinical picture is specifically represented by intrauterine growth retardation without catch-up growth in the first year of life [78]. This deficit is maintained or it gets even worse over time, the adult height being lower than -3DS for average height. At birth, the weight is more impaired than height. The head circumference is normal for age, being in contrast with a lower height, thus the patient has an appearance of macrocephaly. The craniofacial dysmorphias include triangular face, high forehead, micrognathia and down-slanted oral commissures. The limbs are often asymmetrical and a clinodactyly or a camptodactyly of one (fifth finger) or more fingers can be frequently observed. Eating difficulties in infancy, fasting hypoglycemia in infancy and childhood, global developmental delay and cognitive impairments (at about 50% of patients) were also observed. Bone age is retarded, and the radiography also shows a hypoplasia of middle phalanx of fifth finger, which give the appearance of clinodactyly (observed in up to 80% of patients). Sometimes, the patients associate urogenital (hypospadias) or cardiovascular malformations.

2.2.3. Noonan syndrome

This syndrome is very heterogeneous as aetiology, and usually, all the gene mutations described are acting on the signal transduction pathway *RAS/RAF/MEK/ERK* that has a role in regulating cell growth. About 50% of patients have mutations in *PTPN11* gene [79]. An additional percentage of 30% shows mutations in *SOS1* gene and *RAF1* gene. Other gene mutations that lead to Noonan syndrome phenotype are *KRAS*, *NRAS*, *BRAF* and *MAP2K1* [79].

The characteristic features of Noonan syndrome are short stature, craniofacial dysmorphic features, cardiac malformation and thoracic deformity. Short stature has a post-natal onset.

The dysmorphias are represented by triangular face, down-slanted palpebral fissure, hypertelorism, low-set ears and *pterygium colli.* Note that 80% of patients have cardiovascular malformations. The most frequent is pulmonary artery stenosis. About 30% of patients may present hypertrophic cardiomyopathy. Thorax deformation can be *pectus excavatum* or *pectus carinatum.* The patients can associate cryptorchidism (50% of male patients), kidney abnormalities, bleeding disorders, articular hyperlaxity, lymphedema, multiple nevi, hypotonia and epilepsy. The intellectual disability is observed in about 25% of cases.

2.2.4. Cornelia de Lange syndrome

About 50% of patients with Cornelia de Lange syndrome show mutations in *NIPBL* gene [80]. Rarer mutations have been described for *SMC1L1, SMC3* and *RAD21* genes [80].

It is characterized by pre- and post-natal growth retardation, characteristic craniofacial dysmorphic features (narrow forehead with low hair insertion line, synophrys, nostrils anteversion, prognathism, long philtrum, thin lips and down-slanted oral commissures) intellectual disability, upper limbs abnormalities and hypertrichosis. Male patients often present hypospadias and cryptorchidism. Cardiovascular malformations, ophthalmologic abnormalities, deafness, behaviour disorders, global developmental delay, epilepsy and ophthalmologic abnormalities were described. There is a wide phenotypic variability of the syndrome, even some cases with normal IQ have been described.

2.2.5. Rubinstein-Taybi syndrome

This syndrome is also characterized by genetic heterogeneity: *CREBBP* mutation (30–50% of cases), *CREBBP* deletion/ duplication (10–20%), 16p13.3 deletions (including CREBBP) (below 10%) and *EP300* mutation (5%) [81].

Clinically, it is characterized by short stature with post-natal onset, intellectual deficiency, characteristic craniofacial dysmorphia (prominent beaked nose, downslanted palpebral fissures, upper jaw hypoplasia, high arched palate, low-set ears, thin superior lip, microcephaly), and broad thumb with radial angulation, broad hallux, syndactyly, eating difficulties and respiratory disorders in infancy. These patients associate language retardation, hypotonia, cardiac malformations or cryptorchidism.

2.2.6. Prader-Willi syndrome

The Prader-Willi syndrome is the result of paternal loss of imprinted 15q11.2-13 region. This is produced through deletions (70% of cases), uniparental maternal disomy (28%), unbalanced translocations (1%) or mutations in imprinting centre (1%) [82]. Several genes are located in this region, whose function has been already associated with various phenotypic traits of Prader-Willi syndrome (*SNRPN* gene with brain expression, *P* gene with oculocutaneous albinism and *NDN* gene with brain expression) [83].

Most of the clinical specific signs are due to hypothalamic impairment. The clinical presentation is variable, depending on age. Infants with Prader-Willi syndrome show generalized

http://dx.doi.org/10.5772/64561

hypotonia, eating difficulties, males with genital abnormalities (cryptorchidism and scrotal hypoplasia) and motor acquisition delays. After the age of 2, children progressively develop obesity due to hyperphagia. A gradually slowdown in growth, the short stature being often installed before pubertal age and accentuated thereafter by the lack of pubertal growth spurt were also noticed. Most patients also have a deficiency of GH, for which a hormonal treatment is proposed, which also ameliorate the associated metabolic abnormalities. The hypothalamic involvement also induces a hypogonadotropic hypogonadism manifested by cryptorchidism and hypospadias in males or delayed puberty in both sexes, which requires hormonal substitution therapy. Often, the intellectual deficiency is mild. Lifespan is usually influenced by the complications of morbid obesity, often seen in the patients with sleep apnoea, diabetes, atherosclerosis and cardiovascular complications.

2.2.7. *Kabuki syndrome*

The genes involved in Kabuki syndrome are *KDM6A* (Xp11.3) and *KMT2D* (12q13.12) [84].

Clinically, it is characterized by short stature with post-natal onset, global developmental delay/intellectual disability, specific craniofacial dysmorphia (long palpebral fissures, ectropion in the third external region of the upper eyelid, sparse eyebrow in third external region, flattening of the nasal pyramid, large and prominent ears, high arched palate and cleft palate), scoliosis, fifth finger brachydactyly and persistence of finger pads. The associated skeletal abnormalities are spine anomalies, often with vertebral cleft, hip joint abnormalities and fifth finger brachydactyly. Cardiovascular malformations are associated in 50% of cases (Tetralogy of Fallot, atrial septum defects or ventricular septum defects). The characteristic craniofacial dysmorphias, post-natal growth retardation and intellectual disability are among the cardinal manifestations of the disease.

2.2.8. *Williams syndrome*

Williams syndrome is secondary to recurrent deletion in 7q11.23 region comprising elastin gene (*ELN*).

The specific features are craniofacial dysmorphias, cardiovascular malformation, short stature, neuropsychiatric and behavioural disorders, and idiopathic hypercalcemia [85]. Growth retardation is observed in both pre-natal and post-natal periods. The patients often present a delayed bone age and low levels of IGF1. Craniofacial phenotype is represented by stellate iris, periorbital oedema, flattening of nasal pyramid, short nose with anteverted nostrils, long philtrum, macrostomy, thick lips, microdontia, multiple diastema, dental malocclusion and micrognathia. The specific cardiovascular malformation is represented by supravalvular aortic stenosis, seen in more than 80% of patients. Other major arteries stenosis could also be seen. Other frequent signs are hyperacusis, thick voice, articular hyperlaxity, kyphoscoliosis and lordosis. Usually the intellectual disability is moderate, although sometimes, it can be very severe and there are also cases described with IQ in the normal range. These children are hypersociable and hyperactive with attention deficit, often characterized as having a 'cocktail party' personality.

3. Clinical and genetic evaluation in genetic short stature

3.1. Anamnestic data

3.1.1. Personal data

In face of a case with short stature, the anamnesis should be conducted in order to obtain the personal information, normal and pathologic, related to

- **Pre-natal period**: pre-natal echography and data on pregnancy (possible incidents and teratogen exposure).
- **Peri-natal period**: data on birth (possible incidents, type of birth), auxology at birth (weight, length, head circumference), gestational age and data on neo-natal period.
- **Infancy period**: data on nutrition, auxology, psychomotor development and others incidents.
- **Childhood period until the moment of evaluation**: data on growth - previous growth data and growth charts (height, weight, head circumference, body mass index); puberty; age at start of pubertal signs and development of these signs; psychosocial development—school performance, or data on intellectual performance, psychologic and affective status, social environment; nutrition: quantity and quality of different nutriments, particularly vitamin D and calcium intake; and level of physical activities.
- **Data on different diseases or treatment**.
- **History of short stature**: time of onset (pre-natal or post-natal), data on evolution and associated signs.

3.1.2. Familial data

The familial history is also very important, and the evaluation should obtain the data on ethnicity, consanguinity, parental height, tempo of height and puberty for the parents, reproductive history of parents and family, family history on growth disorders, familial short stature, skeletal disorders, endocrine disorders and autoimmunity.

3.2. Physical exam

3.2.1. Growth data

In every evaluation of a patient with short stature, the information on actual auxology are essential and include height, weight, head circumference, body mass index (also in standard deviation to the average) and mid-parental height. These values are put on the growth charts to evaluate the growth pattern that is also compared to midparental height.

To evaluate if the short stature is proportionate or not, the upper-to-lower segment ratio and the arm span will be evaluated. In order to see a possible Madelung deformation, the forearm will also be analysed.

3.2.2. *Other associated signs*

A detailed clinical exam, general and on different organs and systems, is necessary to be associated with auxologic evaluation. At adolescence, the evaluation of the puberty signs should always be attentively assessed.

There are some specific signs associated with short stature, which could give a rapid suggestion for the aetiology and diagnosis (**Table 1**) [86].

Clinical signs	Genetic syndromes
Craniofacial dysmorphy	
Midline face abnormalities: hypotelorism, midline clefting, single median incisor	-Hypophysis abnormalities and GH deficiency
Facial asimetry	-Russell Silver syndrome, 22q11.2 deletion
Elf face	-Williams syndrome
Moon face	-Hypercorticism
Synophrys and hypertrichosis	-Cornelia de Lange syndrome
Short nose and anteverted nostrils	-Smith-Lemli-Opitz syndrome
High arched palate	-SHOX deletion, Turner syndrome, 22q11.2 deletion
Pterygium colli	-Turner syndrome, Noonan syndrome
Tegument and adipose tissue abnormalities	
Multiple nevi	-Turner syndrome, Noonan syndrome
Morbid obesity	-Prader Willi syndrome
Skeletal signs	
Disproportionate short stature	-Skeletal dysplasia
Limbs asymmetry	-Russell-Silver syndrome
Cubitus valgum	-Turner syndrome
Madelung deformity	-SHOX deletion, Turner syndrome
4th and/or 5th brachymetacarpia	-SHOX deletion, Turner syndrome, pseudohypoparathyroidism
Broad thumb	-Rubinstein-Taybi syndrome
5th finger clinodactyly	-Russell Silver syndrome
Cardio-vascular malformation	
Bicuspid aortic valve, aortic coarctation	-Turner syndrome
Supravalvulary aortic stenosis	-Williams syndrome
Pulmonary stenosis	-Noonan syndrome
Urogenital malformation	
Cryptorchidism	-Prader Willi syndrome, Noonan syndrome, Rubinstein Taybi syndrome
Micropenis	-Prader Willi syndrome, congenital GH deficiency
Shawl scrotum	-Aarskog syndrome

Table 1. Clinical signs indicating different genetic syndromes in patients with short stature [86].

Clinical feature	Skeletal dysplasia
Limbs	
Rhizomelic shortening	-achondroplasia, thanatophoric dysplasia, diastrophic dysplasia, spondyloepiphyseal dysplasia (SED)
Mesomelic shortening	-Langer mesomelic dysplasia
Acromelic shortening	-acrodysostosis
Micromelia	-achondrogenesis, Kniest dysplasia, dyssegmental dysplasia
Short trunk	-Kniest syndrome, metatropic dysplasia, SED
Thorax/ribs	
Long or narrow thorax	-Metatropic dysplasia
Pear-shaped chest	-Thanatophoric dysplasia, short-rib polydactyly syndrome
Radial ray defects	-Cornelia de Lange syndrome
Polydactyly	-Chondroectodermal dysplasia, short-rib polydactyly
Hands and feet	
Hitchhiker thumb	-Diastrophic dysplasia
Clubfoot	-Diastrophic dysplasia, Kniest dysplasia, OI
Nails	
Hypoplastic nails	-Chondroectodermal dysplasia
Joints	
Multiple joint dislocations	-Larsen and otopalatodigital syndrome
Long bone fractures	-OI, hypophosphatasia, achondrogenesis type I
Skull	
Macrocephaly	-Achondroplasia, achondrogenesis, thanatophoric dysplasia
Craniosynostosis	-Craniosynostosis syndromes, hypophosphatasia
Cloverleaf skull	-Thanatophoric dysplasia, craniosynostosis
Caput membranaceum	-Hypophosphatasia, osteogenesis imperfecta (OI)
Multiple wormian bones	-Cleidocranial dysplasia, osteogenesis imperfecta
Eyes	
Congenital cataract	-Chondrodysplasia punctata
Myopia	-Kniest dysplasia and spondyloepiphiseal dysplasia
Mouth	
High arched/cleft palate	-Kniest dysplasia, diastrophic dysplasia, metatropic dysplasia
Ears	
Acute swelling of the pinnae	-Diastrophic dysplasia
Heart	
Atrial septal defect	-Chondroectodermal dysplasia
Patent ductus arteriosus	-Lethal short-limbed skeletal dysplasias
Mental retardation	
	-Genetic syndromes—Rubinstein-Taybi syndrome
	-Cranium pathology—craniostenosis
	-Metabolic disorders—lysosomal storage diseases

Table 2. Clinical signs indicating different skeletal dysplasias in patients with short stature [87].

If the patient presents skeletal dysplasia, some clinical signs could orient to the aetiology (**Table 2**) [87].

3.3. Investigations

3.3.1. Imagistic investigations

When evaluating a child with short stature, an X-ray of hand and fist is needed to assess bone age and growth potential. In primary short stature, the bone age is usually not delayed, compared to secondary or idiopathic short stature where a retarded bone age is observed. The bone age is necessary to obtain the predicted height for one patient. This examination is also indicated in parents, if they also have short stature and bone deformities.

If the patient shows clinical signs of skeletal dysplasia, supplementary radiographs are needed to assess long bones, spine and skull, in particular, the forearm (AP), pelvic radiographs (AP), radiographs of the knee (AP) and spine (AP, lateral). Thus, in disproportionate short stature, the radiographs could bring important indicators to establish the diagnosis of the type of skeletal dysplasia, according to the affected area.

Sometimes, at radiography, there are not significant skeletal changes, but even so it cannot rule out skeletal dysplasia, radiological monitoring being required, with repeated radiographs, which may change over time.

3.3.2. Laboratory analysis

Represent the first-line tests indicated in patients with short stature, particularly not elucidated by clinical signs. These analyses must always evaluate the most common causes responsible for somatic developmental delay: anaemic syndrome (erythrocytes, haemoglobin, haematocrit, iron); inflammatory syndrome (erythrocyte sedimentation rate, leucocytes); kidney function and bone metabolism abnormalities (creatinine, urea, sodium, potassium, calcium, magnesium, phosphor and alkaline phosphatase); renal tubular acidosis (acid-base balance); other renal disorders (urinalysis); malabsorption syndrome (iron, ferritin, total protein and albumin); celiac disease (IgA anti-endomysium and anti-transglutaminase, total IgA); hypothyroidism (TSH, T4 free); and growth hormone deficiency (IGF1).

3.4. Genetic testing

Genetic testing follows to the routine non-specific laboratory analysis. It should be performed after an informed consent for genetic testing is obtained. If all the routine tests are negative and clinical examination is not suggestive for certain pathology, a karyotype to any female patient with short stature is routinely indicated. For a male patient with isolated short stature, there is no consensus on routine testing by karyotype; however, an argument in performing the karyotype being to detect a possible syndrome 45,X/46,XY.

If there are no clinical, imagistic or laboratory suggestions for a specific disease, a whole genome analysis of copy number variants by CGH array (array based comparative genomic hybridization) or SNP array (array based single nucleotide polymorphism genotyping) will be indicated. When there is the possibility, an analysis based on massive parallel sequencing technology that will evaluate the whole exome or a panel of genes well known to be implicated in short stature will be proposed. The algorithm of a genetic evaluation in short stature is described in **Figure 1**.

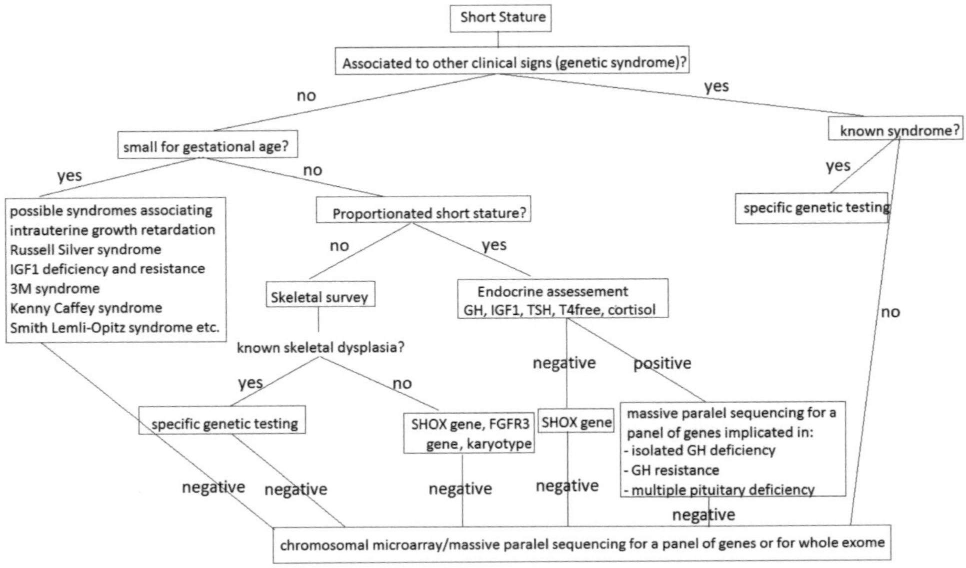

Figure 1. Algorithm for genetic testing in short stature [4, 88].

In a patient with isolated proportioned short stature, the most common causes are numeric abnormalities of X chromosome, SHOX gene mutations, discrete skeletal dysplasia, endocrine disorders, SGA without catch-up growth, constitutional growth retardation and familial short stature. Thus, the genetic testing should take into consideration these aspects.

The patients with SGA without catch-up growth are a special category of patients with short stature, usually proportioned. The majority of patients with SGA (90%) recuperate the deficit by the age of 1, maximum 2 years. Still about 10% of these patients remain with somatic deficit. Often, these patients present associated dysmorphic signs. The main syndromes that have to be taken into consideration in this situation are Russell-Silver syndrome, Bloom syndrome, Nijmegan breakage syndrome, Cockayne syndrome, Dubowitz syndrome, deficit in IGF1, resistance to IGF1, Kenny-Caffey syndrome, Schimke dysplasia or Smith-Lemli-Opitz syndrome [88].

4. Conclusions

Short stature is a strongly genetically determined pathology. The group of genetic disorders with primary effect on growth is very heterogeneous and comprises two important categories

http://dx.doi.org/10.5772/64561

of pathologies: skeletal dysplasia and different genetic syndromes with primary effect on growth. Their diagnosis is often difficult, thus, knowledge of the main clinical signs of each syndrome and the algorithm for clinical diagnosis and genetic testing will practically lead to an easier clinical and etiologic diagnosis.

Acknowledgements

I would like to thank the "Iuliu Hatieganu" University of Medicine and Pharmacy of Cluj-Napoca (Miclea Diana, research grant 4944/24/08.03.2016) for financial support of this book chapter.

Author details

Diana Miclea

Address all correspondence to: bolca12diana@yahoo.com

"Iuliu Hatieganu" University of Medicine and Pharmacy, Dept. of Medical Genetics, Cluj-Napoca, Romania

References

[1] Silventoinen K, Sammalisto S, Perola M, Boomsma DI, Cornes BK, Davis C, et al. Heritability of adult body height: a comparative study of twin cohorts in eight countries. Twin Res. 2003;6(5):399–408. DOI: 10.1375/136905203770326402

[2] Roche AF. Secular trends in human growth, maturation, and development. Monogr Soc Res Child Dev. 1997;44(3–4):1–120.

[3] Ogata T. Genetics of human growth. Clin Pediatr Endocrinol. 2006;15(2):45–53. DOI: 10.1297/cpe.15.45

[4] Dauber A, Rosenfeld RG, Hirschhorn JN. Genetic evaluation of short stature. J Clin Endocrinol Metab. 2014;99(9):3080–3092. DOI: 10.1210/jc.2014-1506

[5] Lango Allen H, Estrada K, Lettre G, Berndt SI, Weedon MN, Rivadeneira F, et al. Hundreds of variants clustered in genomic loci and biological pathways affect human height. Nature. 2010;467(7317):832–838. DOI: 10.1038/nature09410

[6] Weedon MN, Lango H, Lindgren CM, Wallace C, Evans DM, Mangino M, et al. Genome-wide association analysis identifies 20 loci that influence adult height. Nat Genet. 2008;40(5):575–583. DOI: 10.1038/ng.121

[7] Sovio U, Bennett AJ, Millwood IY, Molitor J, O'Reilly PF, Timpson NJ, et al. Genetic determinants of height growth assessed longitudinally from infancy to adulthood in the northern Finland birth cohort 1966. PLoS Genet. 2009;5(3):e1000409. DOI: 10.1371/journal.pgen.1000409

[8] Song KC, Jin SL, Kwon AR, Chae HW, Ahn JM, Kim DH, et al. Etiologies and characteristics of children with chief complaint of short stature. Ann Pediatr Endocrinol Metab. 2015;20(1):34–39. DOI: 10.6065/apem.2015.20.1.34

[9] Flechtner I, Lambot-Juhan K, Teissier R, Colmenares A, Baujat G, Beltrand J, et al. Unexpected high frequency of skeletal dysplasia in idiopathic short stature and small for gestational age patients. Eur J Endocrinol. 2014;170(5):677–684. DOI: 10.1530/EJE-13-0864

[10] Rappold G, Blum WF, Shavrikova EP, Crowe BJ, Roeth R, Quigley CA, et al. Genotypes and phenotypes in children with short stature: clinical indicators of SHOX haploinsufficiency. J Med Genet. 2007;44(5):306–313. DOI: 10.1136/jmg.2006.046581

[11] Warman ML, Cormier-Daire V, Hall C, Krakow D, Lachman R, LeMerrer M, et al. Nosology and classification of genetic skeletal disorders: 2010 revision. Am J Med Genet A. 2011;155A(5):943–968. DOI: 10.1002/ajmg.a.33909

[12] Su N, Jin M, Chen L. Role of FGF/FGFR signaling in skeletal development and homeostasis: learning from mouse models. Bone Res. 2014;2:14003. DOI: 10.1038/boneres.2014.3

[13] Peters K, Ornitz D, Werner S, Williams L. Unique expression pattern of the FGF receptor 3 gene during mouse organogenesis. Dev Biol. 1993;155(2):423–430. DOI: 10.1006/dbio.1993.1040

[14] Shiang R, Thompson LM, Zhu YZ, Church DM, Fielder TJ, Bocian M, et al. Mutations in the transmembrane domain of FGFR3 cause the most common genetic form of dwarfism, achondroplasia. Cell. 1994;78(2):335–342. DOI: 10.1016/0092-8674(94)90302-6

[15] Rousseau F, Bonaventure J, Legeai-Mallet L, Pelet A, Rozet JM, Maroteaux P, et al. Mutations in the gene encoding fibroblast growth factor receptor-3 in achondroplasia. Nature. 1994;371(6494):252–254. DOI: 10.1038/371252a0

[16] Bellus GA, Hefferon TW, Ortiz de Luna RI, Hecht JT, Horton WA, Machado M, et al. Achondroplasia is defined by recurrent G380R mutations of FGFR3. Am J Hum Genet. 1995;56(2):368–373.

[17] Wilkin DJ, Szabo JK, Cameron R, Henderson S, Bellus GA, Mack ML, et al. Mutations in fibroblast growth-factor receptor 3 in sporadic cases of achondroplasia occur exclusively on the paternally derived chromosome. Am J Hum Genet. 1998;63(3):711–716. DOI: 10.1086/302000

[18] Bober MB, Bellus GA, Nikkel SM, Tiller GE. Hypochondroplasia [Internet]. 15/07/1999 [Updated: 26/09/2013]. Available from: www.ncbi.nlm.nih.gov/books/NBK1477/ [Accessed: 02/03/2016]

[19] Mullis PE, Patel MS, Brickell PM, Hindmarsh PC, Brook CG. Growth characteristics and response to growth hormone therapy in patients with hypochondroplasia: genetic linkage of the insulin-like growth factor I gene at chromosome 12q23 to the disease in a subgroup of these patients. Clin Endocrinol (Oxf). 1991;34(4):265–274. DOI: 10.1111/j.1365-2265.1991.tb03765.x

[20] Walker BA, Murdoch JL, McKusick VA, Langer LO, Beals RK. Hypochondroplasia. Am J Dis Child. 1971;122(2):95–104. DOI: 10.1001/archpedi.1971.02110020029001

[21] Bellus GA, Bamshad MJ, Przylepa KA, Dorst J, Lee RR, Hurko O, et al. Severe achondroplasia with developmental delay and acanthosis nigricans (SADDAN): phenotypic analysis of a new skeletal dysplasia caused by a Lys650Met mutation in fibroblast growth factor receptor 3. Am J Med Genet. 1999;85(1):53–65.

[22] Zankl A, Elakis G, Susman RD, Inglis G, Gardener G, Buckley MF, et al. Prenatal and postnatal presentation of severe achondroplasia with developmental delay and acanthosis nigricans (SADDAN) due to the FGFR3 Lys650Met mutation. Am J Med Genet A. 2008;146A(2):212–218. DOI: 10.1002/ajmg.a.32085

[23] Xue Y, Sun A, Mekikian PB, Martin J, Rimoin DL, Lachman RS, et al. FGFR3 mutation frequency in 324 cases from the International Skeletal Dysplasia Registry. Mol Genet Genomic Med. 2014;2(6):497–503. DOI: 10.1002/mgg3.96

[24] Tavormina PL, Shiang R, Thompson LM, Zhu YZ, Wilkin DJ, Lachman RS, et al. Thanatophoric dysplasia (types I and II) caused by distinct mutations in fibroblast growth factor receptor 3. Nat Genet. 1995;9(3):321–328. DOI: 10.1038/ng0395-321

[25] Langer LO, Yang SS, Hall JG, Sommer A, Kottamasu SR, Golabi M, et al. Thanatophoric dysplasia and cloverleaf skull. Am J Med Genet Suppl. 1987;3:167–179. DOI: 10.1002/ajmg.1320280521

[26] Pannier S, Martinovic J, Heuertz S, Delezoide AL, Munnich A, Schibler L, et al. Thanatophoric dysplasia caused by double missense FGFR3 mutations. Am J Med Genet A. 2009;149A(6):1296–1301. DOI: 10.1002/ajmg.a.32880

[27] Shaker JL, Albert C, Fritz J, Harris G. Recent developments in osteogenesis imperfecta. F1000Res. 2015;4(F1000 Faculty Rev):681. DOI: 10.12688/f1000research.6398.1

[28] Exposito JY, Cluzel C, Garrone R, Lethias C. Evolution of collagens. Anat Rec. 2002;268(3):302–316. DOI: 10.1002/ar.10162

[29] Gelse K, Pöschl E, Aigner T. Collagens-structure, function, and biosynthesis. Adv Drug Deliv Rev. 2003;55(12):1531–1546. DOI: 10.1016/j.addr.2003.08.002

[30] Kadler KE, Baldock C, Bella J, Boot-Handford RP. Collagens at a glance. J Cell Sci. 2007;120(Pt 12):1955–1958. DOI: 10.1242/jcs.03453

[31] Sillence DO, Senn A, Danks DM. Genetic heterogeneity in osteogenesis imperfecta. J Med Genet. 1979;16(2):101–116. DOI: 10.1136/jmg.16.2.101

[32] Krakow D, Rimoin DL. The skeletal dysplasias. Genet Med. 2010;12(6):327–341. DOI: 10.1097/GIM.0b013e3181daae9b

[33] Nishimura G, Haga N, Kitoh H, Tanaka Y, Sonoda T, Kitamura M, et al. The phenotypic spectrum of COL2A1 mutations. Hum Mutat. 2005;26(1):36–43. DOI: 10.1002/humu.20179

[34] Chan D, Cole WG, Chow CW, Mundlos S, Bateman JF. A COL2A1 mutation in achondrogenesis type II results in the replacement of type II collagen by type I and III collagens in cartilage. J Biol Chem. 1995;270(4):1747–1753. DOI: 10.1074/jbc.270.4.1747

[35] Godfrey M, Hollister DW. Type II achondrogenesis-hypochondrogenesis: identification of abnormal type II collagen. Am J Med Genet. 1988;43(6):904–913.

[36] Wynne-Davies R, Hall C. Two clinical variants of spondylo-epiphysial dysplasia congenita. J Bone Joint Surg Br. 1982;64(4):435–441.

[37] Gilbert-Barnes E, Langer LO, Opitz JM, Laxova R, Sotelo-Arila C. Kniest dysplasia: radiologic, histopathological, and scanning electronmicroscopic findings. Am J Med Genet. 1996;63(1):34–45. DOI: 10.1002/(SICI)1096-8628(19960503)

[38] Snead MP, Yates JRW. Clinical and molecular genetics of Stickler syndrome. J Med Genet. 1999;36(5):353–359. DOI: 10.1136/jmg.36.5.353

[39] Robin NH, Moran RT, Ala-Kokko L. Stickler Syndrome [Internet]. 09/06/2000 [Updated: 26/11/2014]. Available from: www.ncbi.nlm.nih.gov/books/NBK1302 [Accessed: 02/03/2016]

[40] Holden P, Meadows R S, Chapman KL, Grant ME, Kadler KE, Briggs MD. Cartilage oligomeric matrix protein interacts with type IX collagen, and disruptions to these interactions identify a pathogenetic mechanism in a bone dysplasia family. J Biol Chem. 2001;276(8):6046–6055. DOI: 10.1074/jbc.M009507200

[41] Hecht JT, Hayes E, Haynes R, Cole WG. COMP mutations, chondrocyte function and cartilage matrix. Matrix Biol. 2005;23(8):525–533. DOI: 10.1016/j.matbio.2004.09.006

[42] Unger SL, Briggs MD, Holden P, Zabel B, Ala-Kokko L, Paassilta P, et al. Multiple epiphyseal dysplasia: radiographic abnormalities correlated with genotype. Pediatr Radiol. 2001;31(1):10–18. DOI: 10.1007/s002470000362

[43] Unger S, Hecht JT. Pseudoachondroplasia and multiple epiphyseal dysplasia: new etiologic developments. Am J Med Genet. 2001;106(4):244–250. DOI: 10.1002/ajmg.10234

[44] Seo SG, Song H-R, Kim HW, Yoo WJ, Shim JS, Chung CY, et al. Comparison of orthopaedic manifestations of multiple epiphyseal dysplasia caused by MATN3 versus COMP mutations: a case control study. BMC Musculoskelet Disord. 2014;15:84. DOI: 10.1186/1471-2474-15-84

[45] Shen G. The role of type X collagen in facilitating and regulating endochondral ossification of articular cartilage. Orthod Craniofac Res. 2005;8(1):11–17. DOI: 10.1111/j.1601-6343.2004.00308.x

[46] Poulson AV, Hooymans JMM, Richards AJ, Bearcroft P, Murthy R, Baguley DM, et al. Clinical features of type 2 Stickler syndrome. J Med Genet. 2004;41(8):e107. DOI: 10.1136/jmg.2004.018382

[47] Rose PS, Ahn NU, Levy HP, Magid D, Davis J, Liberfarb RM, et al. The hip in Stickler syndrome. J Pediatr Orthop. 2001;21(5):657–663. DOI: 10.1097/01241398-200109000-00020

[48] Rose PS, Ahn NU, Levy HP, Ahn UM, Davis J, Liberfarb RM, et al. Thoracolumbar spinal abnormalities in Stickler syndrome. Spine. 2001;26(4):403–409. DOI: 10.1097/00007632-200102150-00017

[49] Harel T, Rabinowitz R, Hendler N, Galil A, Flusser H, Chemke J, et al. COL11A2 mutation associated with autosomal recessive Weissenbacher-Zweymuller syndrome: molecular and clinical overlap with otospondylomegaepiphyseal dysplasia (OSMED). Am J Med Genet A. 2005;132A(1):33–35. DOI: 10.1002/ajmg.a.30371

[50] Hästbacka J, de la Chapelle A, Mahtani MM, Clines G, Reeve-Daly MP, Daly M, et al. The diastrophic dysplasia gene encodes a novel sulfate transporter: positional cloning by fine-structure linkage disequilibrium mapping. Cell. 1994;78(6):1073–1087. DOI: 10.1016/0092-8674(94)90281-X

[51] Ayoubi JM, Jouk PS, Pons JC. Diastrophic dwarfism and pregnancy. Lancet. 2001;358(9295):1778. DOI: 10.1016/S0140-6736(01)06806-4

[52] Bonafe L, Mittaz-Crettol L, Ballhausen D, Superti-Furga A. Diastrophic Dysplasia [Internet]. 15/11/2004 [Updated: 18/07/2013]. Available from: www.ncbi.nlm.nih.gov/books/NBK1350 [Accessed: 02/03/2016]

[53] Aleck KA, Grix A, Clericuzio C, Kaplan P, Adomian GE, Lachman R, et al. Dyssegmental dysplasias: clinical, radiographic, and morphologic evidence of heterogeneity. Am J Med Genet. 1987;27(2):295–312. DOI: 10.1002/ajmg.1320270208

[54] Rieubland C, Jacquemont S, Mittaz L, Osterheld M-C, Vial Y, Superti-Furga A, et al. Phenotypic and molecular characterization of a novel case of dyssegmental dysplasia, Silverman-Handmaker type. Eur J Med Genet. 2010;53(5):294–298. DOI: 10.1016/j.ejmg.2010.06.005

[55] Stum M, Davoine CS, Fontaine B, Nicole S. Schwartz-Jampel syndrome and perlecan deficiency. Acta Myol. 2005;24(2):89–92.

[56] Spranger J, Hall BD, Häne B, Srivastava A, Stevenson RE. Spectrum of Schwartz-Jampel syndrome includes micromelic chondrodysplasia, kyphomelic dysplasia, and Burton disease. Am J Med Genet. 2000;94(4):287–295. DOI: 10.1002/1096-8628(20001002)94:4<287::AID-AJMG5>3.0.CO;2-G

[57] Kiani C, Chen L, Wu YJ, Yee AJ, Yang BB. Structure and function of aggrecan. Cell Res. 2002;12(1):19–32. DOI: 10.1038/sj.cr.7290106

[58] Anderson IJ, Tsipouras P, Scher C, Ramesar RS, Martell RW, Beighton P. Spondyloepiphyseal dysplasia, mild autosomal dominant type is not due to primary defects of type II collagen. Am J Med Genet. 1990;37(2):272–276. DOI: 10.1002/ajmg.1320370223

[59] Masuyama R, Vriens J, Voets T, Karashima Y, Owsianik G, Vennekens R, et al. TRPV4-mediated calcium influx regulates terminal differentiation of osteoclasts. Cell Metab. 2008;8(3):257–265. DOI: 10.1016/j.cmet.2008.08.002

[60] Geneviève D, Le Merrer M, Feingold J, Munnich A, Maroteaux P, Cormier-Daire V. Revisiting metatropic dysplasia: presentation of a series of 19 novel patients and review of the literature. Am J Med Genet A. 2008;146A(8):992–996. DOI: 10.1002/ajmg.a.32191

[61] Munns CJF, Haase HR, Crowther LM, Hayes MT, Blaschke R, Rappold G, et al. Expression of SHOX in human fetal and childhood growth plate. J Clin Endocrinol Metab. 2004;89(8):4130–4135. DOI: 10.1210/jc.2003-032230

[62] Marchini A, Marttila T, Winter A, Caldeira S, Malanchi I, Blaschke RJ, et al. The short stature homeodomain protein SHOX induces cellular growth arrest and apoptosis and is expressed in human growth plate chondrocytes. J Biol Chem. 2004:279(35):37103–37114. DOI: 10.1074/jbc.M307006200

[63] Rao E, Weiss B, Fukami M, Rump A, Niesler B, Mertz A, et al. Pseudoautosomal deletions encompassing a novel homeobox gene cause growth failure in idiopathic short stature and Turner syndrome. Nat Genet. 1997:16(1):54–63. DOI: 10.1038/ng0597-54

[64] Rappold GA, Fukami M, Niesler B, Schiller S, Zumkeller W, Bettendorf M, et al. Deletions of the homeobox gene SHOX (short stature homeobox) are an important cause of growth failure in children with short stature. J Clin Endocrinol Metab. 2002;87(3):1402–1406. DOI: 10.1210/jcem.87.3.8328

[65] Stuppia L. SHOX mutations detected by FISH and direct sequencing in patients with short stature. J Med Genet. 2003;40(2):e11. DOI: 10.1136/jmg.40.2.e11

[66] Hintz RL. SHOX mutations. Rev Endocr Metab Disord. 2002;3(4):363–367.

[67] Leka SK, Kitsiou-Tzeli S, Kalpini-Mavrou A, Kanavakis E. Short stature and dysmorphology associated with defects in the SHOX gene. Hormones (Athens). 2006;5(2):107–118.

[68] Ogata T. SHOX haploinsufficiency: lessons from clinical studies. Curr Opin Endocrinol Diabetes. 2002;9(1):13–20. DOI: 10.1097/00060793-200202000-00003

[69] Elsheikh M, Dunger DB, Conway GS, Wass JAH. Turner's syndrome in adulthood. Endocr Rev. 2002;23(1):120–140. DOI: 10.1210/edrv.23.1.0457

[70] Cabrol S. Turner syndrome. Ann Endocrinol (Paris). 2007;68(1):2–9. DOI: 10.1016/j.ando.2006.12.002

[71] Sybert VP, McCauley E. Turner's syndrome. N Engl J Med. 2004;351(12):1227–38. DOI: 10.1056/NEJMra030360

[72] Migeon BR, Luo S, Jani M, Jeppesen P. The severe phenotype of females with tiny ring X chromosomes is associated with inability of these chromosomes to undergo X inactivation. Am J Hum Genet. 1994;55(3):497–504.

[73] Fuke T, Mizuno S, Nagai T, Hasegawa T, Horikawa R, Miyoshi Y, et al. Molecular and clinical studies in 138 Japanese patients with Silver-Russell syndrome. PLoS One. 2013;8(3):e60105. DOI: 10.1371/journal.pone.0060105

[74] Eggermann T. Russell-Silver syndrome. Am J Med Genet C Semin Med Genet. 2010;154C(3):355–364. DOI: 10.1002/ajmg.c.30274

[75] Dörr S, Midro AT, Färber C, Giannakudis J, Hansmann I. Construction of a detailed physical and transcript map of the candidate region for Russell-Silver syndrome on chromosome 17q23-q24. Genomics. 2001;71(2):174–181. DOI: 10.1006/geno.2000.6413

[76] van Haelst MM, Eussen HJFMM, Visscher F, de Ruijter JLM, Drop SLS Lindhout D, et al. Silver-Russell phenotype in a patient with pure trisomy 1q32.1-q42.1: further delineation of the pure 1q trisomy syndrome. J Med Genet. 2002;39(8): 582–585. DOI: 10.1136/jmg.39.8.582

[77] Li CC, Chodirker BN, Dawson AJ, Chudley AE. Severe hemihypotrophy in a female infant with mosaic Turner syndrome: a variant of Russell-Silver syndrome? Clin Dysmorphol. 2004;13(2):95–98. DOI: 10.1097/00019605-200404000-00008

[78] Price SM, Stanhope R, Garrett C, Preece MA, Trembath RC. The spectrum of Silver-Russell syndrome: a clinical and molecular genetic study and new diagnostic criteria. J Med Genet. 1999;36(11):837–842. DOI: 10.1136/jmg.36.11.837

[79] Ferrero GB, Baldassarre G, Delmonaco AG, Biamino E, Banaudi E, Carta C, et al. Clinical and molecular characterization of 40 patients with Noonan syndrome. Eur J Med Genet. 2008;51(6):566–572. DOI: 10.1016/j.ejmg.2008.06.011

[80] Ramos FJ, Puisac B, Baquero-Montoya C, Gil-Rodríguez MC, Bueno I, Deardorff MA, et al. Clinical utility gene card for: Cornelia de Lange syndrome. Eur J Hum Genet. 2015;23(10):1431. DOI: 10.1038/ejhg.2014.270

[81] Milani D, Manzoni FMP, Pezzani L, Ajmone P, Gervasini C, Menni F, et al. Rubinstein-Taybi syndrome: clinical features, genetic basis, diagnosis, and management. Ital J Pediatr. 2015;41:4. DOI: 10.1186/s13052-015-0110-1

[82] Driscoll DJ, Miller JL, Schwartz S, Cassidy SB. Prader-Willi Syndrome [Internet]. 06/10/1998 [Updated: 04/02/2016]. Available from: www.ncbi.nih.gov/books/NBK1330/ [Accessed: 02/03/2016]

[83] MacDonald HR, Wevrick R. The necdin gene is deleted in Prader-Willi syndrome and is imprinted in human and mouse. Hum Mol Genet. 1997;6(11):1873–1878. DOI: 10.1093/hmg/6.11.1873

[84] Arnaud M, Barat-Houari M, Gatinois V, Sanchez E, Lyonnet S, Touitou I, et al. Kabuki syndrome: update and review. Arch Pediatr. 2015;22(6):653–660. DOI: 10.1016/j.arcped.2015.03.020

[85] Pober BR. Williams-Beuren syndrome. N Engl J Med. 2010;362(3):239–252. DOI: 10.1056/NEJMra0903074

[86] Oostdijk W, Grote FK, de Muinck Keizer-Schrama SMPF, Wit JM. Diagnostic approach in children with short stature. Horm Res. 2009;72(4):206–217. DOI: 10.1159/000236082

[87] Chen H. Skeletal Dysplasia [Internet]. [Updated: 02/03/2015]. Available from: emedicine.medscape.com/article/943343-clinical#b4 [Accessed: 02/03/2016]

[88] Seaver LH, Irons M. ACMG practice guideline: genetic evaluation of short stature. Genet Med. 2009;11(6):465–470. DOI: 10.1097/GIM.0b013e3181a7e8f8

Section 3

Signaling Pathways and Molecular Mechanisms of Restricted Growth

Chapter 4

Molecular Defects and Cellular Dysfunctions in Restricted Growth Conditions

Monica Mottes and Patricia Marie-Jeanne Lievens

Additional information is available at the end of the chapter

http://dx.doi.org/10.5772/64560

Abstract

Restricted growth (RG) or dwarfism is a varied phenotype ascribable to many different causes, most of which are genetic. Conditions associated with disproportionate short stature (DSS) are usually caused by *de novo* dominant mutations in genes coding for proteins involved in cartilage/bone development. Rarer conditions, which may occur in inbred families, show an autosomal recessive inheritance. Causative mutations, consequent to cellular dysfunctions, genotype-to-phenotype correlations in RG conditions such as achondroplasia, hypochondroplasia, thanatophoric dysplasia, severe achondroplasia with delay in development and acanthosis nigricans, pseudoachondroplasia, multiple epiphyseal dysplasia, diastrophic dysplasia, achondrogenesis, and osteogenesis imperfecta, are discussed in this chapter.

Keywords: dwarfism, cartilage, bone, chondrocyte, osteoblast

1. Introduction

Human height is a genetically complex phenotype. In recent years, several genome-wide association studies (GWAS) have collectively identified hundreds of common variants with a putative effect on determining adult height [1]. The variability between individuals has a normal distribution; extremes in height are often caused by monogenic mutations in genes involved in growth control. Gain in height in children is determined by the rate of endochondral ossification, i.e. the rate of proliferation of chondrocytes at the growth plate, a thin layer of cartilage that is found in most bones, other than skull and facial bones. Newly generated cartilage tissue is remodeled into bone tissue; as new bone is progressively created at the growth plate, bones grow longer and children grow taller. At puberty increasing levels of estrogen, in both females and males, lead to increased apoptosis of chondrocytes in the growth plate; growth slows down and later stops when the entire cartilage has become replaced by bone, leaving only a thin epiphyseal scar. Systemic factors such as growth and thyroid hormones provide important signals for the regulation of cartilage/bone growth by modulating expression of locally produced factors, such as tissue-specific transcription factors (e.g. short stature homeobox-containing factor, SHOX), multiple fibroblast growth factors (FGFs), bone morphogenetic proteins (BMPs), secreted signaling factors such as Wnts, and many others. Cartilage extracellular matrix components, secreted by chondrocytes, also play a crucial role in regulating growth plate activity. Dysfunctions in any of the multiple players in this complex process may cause genetic growth disorders. Gene mutations affecting various stages of the bone formation process, e.g. osteoblast differentiation, bone extracellular matrix deposition and mineralization, may as well result in substantial growth deficiency, a hallmark feature of osteogenesis imperfecta, a molecularly heterogeneous group of connective tissue disorders.

In this chapter, we will describe some paradigmatic conditions of restricted growth from the cell biologist's perspective. We will first consider various *cartilage disorders* and then some *bone disorders*. Our approach will start from the description of gene defects, the cellular dysfunctions they cause, their consequences on the extracellular matrix, and finally we will describe briefly the associated phenotypes, trying to compare, whenever possible, similar conditions.

2. Cartilage disorders associated with impaired height

Chondrodysplasias causing dwarfism comprise a group of skeletal disorders associated with improper regulation of cartilage growth during endochondral ossification (see **Figure 1** for a

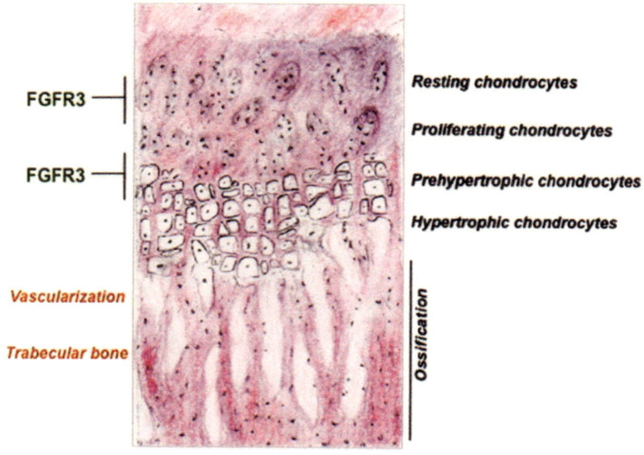

Figure 1. Endochondral ossification. Bone elongation is a tightly regulated process leading to the formation of a cartilage template subsequently replaced by bone. During the process, resting chondrocytes of the growth plates mature into proliferating chondrocytes, which in turn differentiate into prehypertrophic and then hypertrophic chondrocytes. The latter die by apoptosis and are replaced by trabecular bone, as a result of the following vascularization and ossification processes. FGFR3 plays a key role as negative regulator of chondrocytes proliferation and differentiation.

simplified sketch of the process). Although this notion had been widely accepted for a long time, the idea that morphological assessment of the growth plate could be used to distinguish among the different disorders was successfully proposed only in the 1970s [2]. This brought to the concept of "chondrodysplasia families" formulated in the 1980s and the hypothesis that chondrodysplasias that look similar could be pathogenetically related. But it was only in the 1990s, with the advent of molecular genetics identifying the mutated genes associated with different chondrodysplasias, that in many instances chondrodysplasia family disorders turned out to be caused by mutations within the same gene, indeed [3].

2.1. FGFR signaling defects

Dwarf-associated chondrodysplasias are caused by genetic alterations in the *Fibroblast Growth Factor* (*FGF*) *Receptor 3* (*FGFR3*) gene and include achondroplasia (ACH), hypochondroplasia (HCH), thanatophoric dysplasia types I and II (TDI and TDII), and SADDAN [4]. A summary of the most recurrent mutations is shown in **Figure 2**. FGFR3 is a tyrosine kinase highly expressed in the resting and proliferating chondrocyte zones, where it plays key roles in controlling chondrocyte proliferation and/or subsequent cell cycle exit leading to differentiation into prehypertrophic chondrocytes. The transient pool of prehypertrophic chondrocytes will progress into hypertrophy generating an expansive strength required for bone elongation. Hypertrophic chondrocytes will eventually die by apoptosis or differentiate into trabecular osteoblasts allowing bone formation. Several signaling effectors fine-tune the transition from resting to hypertrophic chondrocytes, among which are FGFs. FGF family comprises secreted

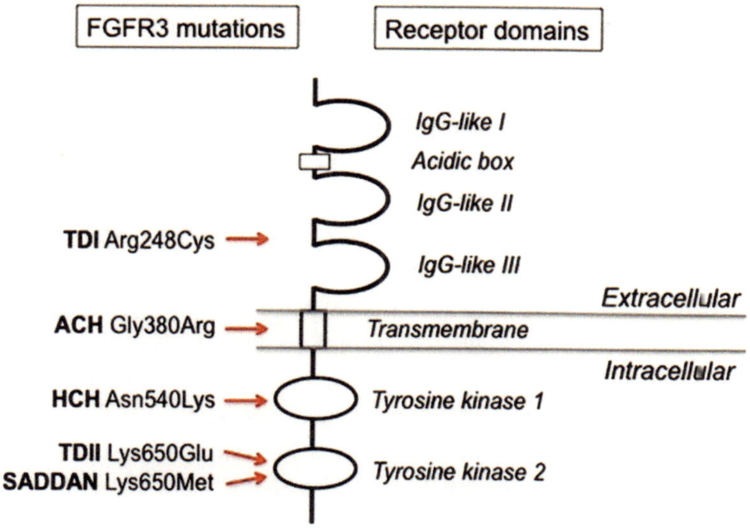

Figure 2. Recurrent FGFR3 mutations in chondrodysplasia. FGFR3 is a tyrosine kinase receptor composed by three IgG-like domains and an acidic box in the extracellular space, a transmembrane domain and two intracellular tyrosine kinase domains. TDI, ACH, HCH, TDII, and SADDAN diseases are caused by point mutations affecting different protein domains. Red arrows indicate where the most recurrent mutations associated with each different chondrodysplasia fall in FGFR3 molecule.

proteins that bind and activate FGFR3 as specific ligands and key roles in endochondral ossification have been attributed to FGF9 and FGF18 [5]. In the presence of heparin or heparan sulfates, FGFs bind to FGFR3 inducing receptor dimerization and subsequent autophosphorylation, which represent the activated state of FGFR3. Once stimulated, FGFR3 molecules trigger the activation of the RAS-MAPK and PLCγ intracellular signaling pathway or—depending on the cell type—of the PI3K or STAT pathways [3]. The mentioned signaling pathways have been shown to regulate several processes including cell proliferation and differentiation and can be activated by other members of the FGFR family (FGFR1, FGFR2, and FGFR4). However, unlike FGFR1, -2, and -4, FGFR3 uses those pathways to negatively regulate bone elongation, as proved by gene ablation in a mouse model resulting in extra-long bones [6]. Further supporting this notion is the recent identification of a missense impairing mutation (Arg621His) in FGFR3 that causes CATSHL (Online Mendelian Inheritance in Man, OMIM #610474) syndrome in humans, also characterized by extra-long bones [7]. A critical step in FGFR function is represented by receptor activity attenuation, a process required to avoid excessive signaling duration. Dwarfism-associated chondrodysplasias are all characterized by gain-of-function mutations that render FGFR3 constitutively active, but with graded levels of signaling potential [4].

Achondroplasia (*ACH*, OMIM #100800) is the most common among human chondrodysplasias and occurs with an incidence of 1:10–30,000 live births. Average adult male height is 131 cm, while average adult female height is 123 cm. Affected newborn infants present with disproportionate shortening of the limbs, a long and narrow trunk, a large skull with frontal bossing, a hypoplastic midface and exaggerated lumbar lordosis, as major clinical features [8]. Skeletal X-rays reveal characteristic abnormalities in the long bones of the limbs, which appear short. This form of dwarfism is caused by point mutations in FGFR3 characterized by autosomal dominant inheritance, as first discovered in the 1990s when heterozygous mutations were mapped to FGFR3 locus on chromosome 4. Almost all patients with typical achondroplasia features bear a glycine-to-arginine substitution at position 380 (Gly380Arg) in FGFR3, resulting from a spontaneous mutation to non achondroplastic parents (primarily fathers), in more than 80% of cases. This conversion shows the highest rate of occurrence among the known genetic germline substitutions, and a correlation with paternal age had been made [9]. FGFR3 protein is composed by an extracellular ligand-binding domain, a transmembrane domain, and an intracellular split tyrosine kinase domain (**Figure 2**). The Gly380Arg mutation falls in the transmembrane region causing a gain in receptor function, which reduces growth plate activity. Transgenic mice models for ACH (see Section Methods) allowed the characterization of FGFR3 function during skeletal development and postnatal growth, via analysis of the consequences derived from the mutation. Cartilage overexpression of FGFR3 bearing the achondroplasia mutation produced small mice with short bones resembling those seen in human achondroplasia. Studies coming from these mice led to postulate a defect in chondrocyte proliferation and/or differentiation, histologically giving rise to a disorganized growth plate [10].

FGFR3 is highly expressed in both proliferating and prehypertrophic chondrocytes where it normally limits their growth rate (**Figure 1**). At the molecular level, the FGFR3-Gly380Arg mutant showed ligand-independent activation and a specific defect in receptor down-regulation resulting in prolonged signaling activity [11]. Interestingly, cartilage targeted overexpression of a ligand (FGF9) that activates FGFR3 also generated a dwarf mouse [12]. These evidences established that FGFR3 signaling negatively regulates bone growth. Among the signaling effectors downstream to FGFR3 activation, STAT and MAPK signals have been the most studied in relation to skeletal development (a scheme of major FGFR3 signaling pathways is presented in **Figure 3**). FGFR3 is thought to inhibit chondrocyte proliferation through the cyclin-dependent kinase inhibitor p21 (WAF1/CIP1), where the latter controls chondrocyte proliferation and terminal differentiation through the recruitment of p38 and ERK effectors [8, 13]. Biochemically, replacement of glycine 380 with arginine causes ligand-independent activation of FGFR3, which increases the constitutive level of phosphotyrosine on FGFR3 [14]. The consequent unregulated signal transduction through FGFR3 impacts growth plate function and therefore long bone development. Several approaches to reduce FGFR3 signaling by blocking receptor activation or inhibiting downstream signals have been proposed. The most promising utilizes an analog of C-type natriuretic peptide (CNP), which antagonizes the mitogen-activated protein (MAP) kinase pathway downstream of the FGFR3 receptor [15].

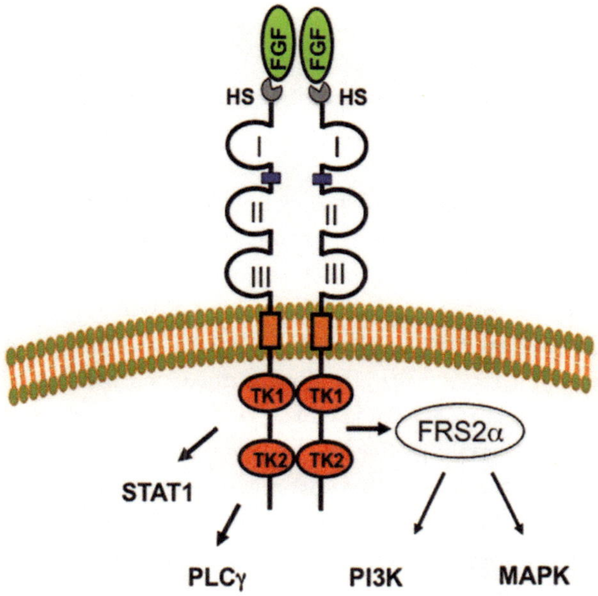

Figure 3. Signaling pathways downstream to FGFR3. Upon binding to specific FGF ligands and heparan sulfates (HS), FGFR3 undergoes dimerization, which causes conformational changes leading to tyrosine autophosphorylation. In this state, the receptor is active and engenders intracellular signal transduction by recruiting specific downstream effectors. STATs and MAPK signaling pathways play key roles in regulating the growth plate function.

Hypochondroplasia (*HCH*, OMIM #146000) shows skeletal features similar to but milder than those seen in ACH, whose differences can be distinguished on clinical and radiographic grounds. Key features are short-limbed dwarfism, lumbar lordosis, stocky build, short and broad bones, and macrocephaly. Adult height ranges between 128 and 165 cm; 2.3 SD below the mean in children, but in some cases stature appears normal. The incidence of HCH is not precisely known, but it is believed to be about as common as ACH. Based on the clinical report of a peculiar case, allelism of HCH and ACH genes was suggested [16]. Subsequent genetic analyses indicated the Asn540Lys substitution in FGFR3, as the most recurrent mutation in HCH patients. The Asn540Lys mutation is inherited in an autosomal dominant manner and accounts for about 60–65% of cases, according to the clinical heterogeneity observed for this disease [17]. Although the amino acid change is semi-conservative, it occurs in a very conserved region of the tyrosine kinase 1 domain. The Asn540Lys mutation favors FGFR3 dimerization determining a gain of function associated with a mild but constitutive autophosphorylation. The lower degree of tyrosine phosphorylation of FGFR3-HCH compared to FGFR3-ACH was correlated with a milder clinical phenotype.

Thanatophoric dysplasia (*TDI*, OMIM #187600) and TDII (OMIM #187601). TDI is a severe autosomal dominant skeletal disorder that is lethal in the neonatal period of life. Two clinically defined TD subtypes have been classified: type I (TDI), characterized by micromelia with bowed femurs and, occasionally, by the presence of cloverleaf skull deformity of varying severity, and type II (TDII) characterized by micromelia with straight femurs and a moderate-to-severe cloverleaf skull deformity. TDI, which is more common, originates from several amino acid substitutions in extracellular and intracellular domains of FGFR3 protein, such as Arg248Cys, Tyr373Cys, and diverse substitutions of the natural stop codon in sense codons, such as X807Gly, X807Arg, and X807Cys, which result in the elongation of FGFR3 protein at the C-terminus by 141 amino acids. Conversely, only the Lys650Glu mutation located in activation loop of the kinase domain of FGFR3 has been associated with TDII [18]. The estimated birth incidence is approximately 1/20,000–1/50,000 being more frequent for TDI than for TDII. Most individuals with TD die within the first few hours or days of life by respiratory insufficiency secondary to reduced thoracic capacity or compression of the brainstem. Several mutations causing TDI lead to constitutive dimerization of FGFR3 due to the introduction of novel cysteines as it is the case for the Arg248Cys mutation, one of the most recurrent ones. Differently, TDII-associated Lys650Glu mutation induces a strong and constitutive ligand-independent tyrosine phosphorylation of FGFR3. This causes the recruitment and activation of several downstream key signaling effectors, among which are members of the STAT family, as shown in cell culture systems, human fetuses, and in a mouse model [19]. Moreover, the constitutive tyrosine phosphorylation acquired by the FGFR3-TDII receptor causes its accumulation within the endoplasmic reticulum (ER)/Golgi compartments impairing receptor trafficking toward the plasma membrane [20].

Severe achondroplasia with delay in development and acanthosis nigricans (*SADDAN*, OMIM #616482). SADDAN is a very rare skeletal disease: only few cases have been described. It clinically resembles TDI, but most of the SADDAN patients survive the perinatal period. This syndrome is additionally characterized by severe neurologic impairments, especially in long survivors and by the development of extensive areas of acanthosis nigricans [21]. SADDAN is caused by a heterozygous mutation in FGFR3 changing lysine 650 in methionine (Lys650Met). Of interest is the observation that the same lysine, when mutated into glutamic acid, gives rise to TDII. A mouse model for the SADDAN disease (see the methods section) highlighted milder long bone abnormalities than in the TDII mouse model, and overgrowth of the cartilaginous tissues was observed in the rib cartilage, trachea, and nasal septum. The presence of the Lys650Met mutation causes the highest constitutive tyrosine phosphorylation among the ligand-independently activated mutant FGFR3 associated with chondrodysplasia. Analogously to FGFR3-TDII, in cell culture models, the SADDAN mutant triggers the activation of several signal transduction effectors from the ER/Golgi, where it is kept due to its premature tyrosine kinase activation [22]. Although all FGFR3-related skeletal dyplasias manifest with profound shortening of the long bones, the phenotypic severity ranges from relatively mild HCH to neonatal lethal TD, where the degree of severity correlates with the degree of activated FGFR3. The different mutations activate FGFR3 and correspondingly inhibit chondrocyte proliferation to different levels when compared to wild-type (wt) FGFR3, with a relative strength being [4]:

$$\text{wt} < \text{Arg540Lys}(\text{HCH}) < \text{Gly380Arg}\ (\text{ACH}) \ll \text{Arg248Cys}(\text{TDI}) = \text{Tyr373Cys}\ \leq \text{Lys650Glu}\ (\text{TDII}).$$

2.2. COMP defects

Thrombospondin-5, better known as cartilage oligomeric protein (*COMP*), is a pentameric extracellular matrix (ECM) protein primarily expressed in chondrocytes and musculoskeletal tissues [23]. Each monomer comprises four domains (**Figure 4**). COMP interacts with several ECM proteins, including collagen II, collagen IX, matrilins, proteoglycans, and others. Through these interactions, COMP plays an important role in matrix assembly. Gene mutations affecting the structure of COMP pentamers cause two different skeletal dysplasias with autosomal dominant inheritance: pseudoachondroplasia (*PSACH*) and multiple epiphyseal dysplasia type 1 (*EDM1*)

PSACH (OMIM #177170) is a disproportionate dwarfing condition with involvement of the long bones, spine, and joints (incidence=1:20.000). Unlike ACH, it is not recognizable at birth: PSACH newborns are normal. Growth retardation is seldom recognized until the second year of life or later, at which time the body proportions resemble those of persons with achondroplasia, but the head circumference and facies are normal. Average adult male height is 120 cm; average adult female height is 116 cm. Radiographic findings of PSACH are distinctive, and another distinctive finding consists of significantly low COMP plasma levels. Scoliosis and lumbar lordosis are common spine abnormalities; osteoarthritis develops by the second/third decade of life affecting all joints. *Molecular pathology—In vitro* studies on human cells and analysis of mouse PSACH models demonstrated that pseudoachondroplasia is an endoplasmic reticulum storage disease, caused by improper folding of mutant COMP. Many causative mutations have been described: they produce either single amino acid substitutions or deletions and cluster in the highly conserved type 3 (Calcium binding) repeat domain TSP 3 (depicted in color pink in the diagram; **Figure 4**). A recurrent mutation in which aspartic acid 469 is deleted (D469 del) accounts for 30% of PSACH cases. All PSACH mutations exert a dominant-negative effect: pentamers composed of both structurally abnormal and normal subunits are retained within the endoplasmic reticulum (ER), promoting an excessive ER stress response and ultimately premature chondrocyte death [24]. The growth failure of patients with PSACH may be explained by an increased death rate of growth-plate chondrocytes. The observation that COMP-deficient mice are not dwarfed and show a normal skeletal phenotype suggested that loss of COMP in the cartilage ECM *per se* is not the primary defect in PSACH [25].

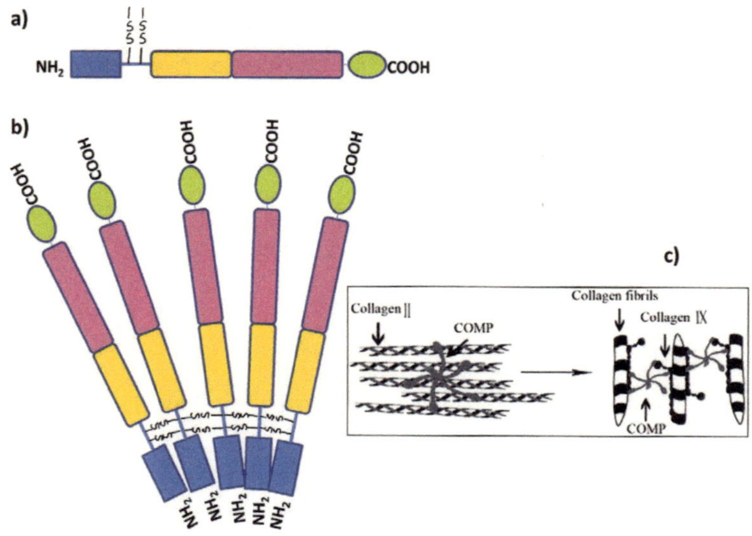

Figure 4. COMP structure and function in the ECM. (a) Schematic representation of COMP monomer, which comprises four domains: An N-terminal pentamerization domain (blue), an EGF-like domain (orange), a highly conserved TSP3 (calcium binding) domain (pink), a C-terminal globular domain (green). (b) COMP oligomer made of five identical disulfide-linked monomers. (c) Schematic representation of COMP interactions with collagens II and IX in cartilage ECM (Open-i nlm.nih.gov).

Epiphyseal dysplasia multiple 1 (*EDM1*, OMIM #132400) is a skeletal dysplasia characterized by mildly impaired height and early onset osteoarthrosis. Due to genetic heterogeneity (defects in other genes may cause similar phenotypes), only 38% of multiple epiphyseal dysplasia (*MED*) spectrum can be ascribed to COMP mutations. MED patients with COMP mutations can be recognized because of significantly low COMP plasma levels. Causative mutations are amino acid substitutions clustered in TSP3 domain; therefore, a phenotypic overlap between PSACH and EDM1 can be observed. However, missense mutations resulting in MED or mild PSACH phenotypes have been described also in the C-terminal domain of COMP (depicted in color green in the diagram; **Figure 4**).

2.3. Sulfate transporter defects

A group of chondrodysplasias showing moderate to lethal phenotypes have been associated with mutations in SLC26A2 gene, which codes for a sulfate-chloride transmembrane exchanger, DTSTD. This protein is predominantly present in chondrocytes, and it ensures proper sulfation of proteoglycans, essential components of the cartilage extracellular matrix. The highly organized structure of cartilage ECM is of crucial importance for the endochondral ossification process. Furthermore, sulfated proteoglycans are important for transmission of FGF signaling [26]. In humans, as well as in animal models, impaired sulfation of proteoglycans due to DTDST gene defects causes a continuous phenotypic spectrum of skeletal dysplasia. The clinical phenotype is modulated by the degree of residual protein activity, as shown in **Figure 5**. All conditions are recessively inherited; heterozygous carriers appear to be asymptomatic [27].

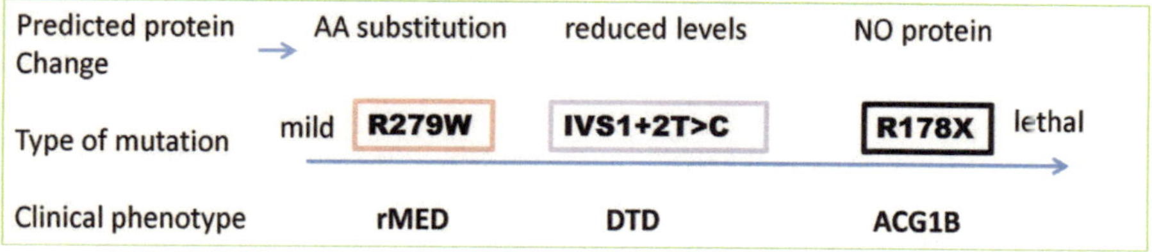

Figure 5. Schematic representation of genotype-to-phenotype correlations along the spectrum of SLC26A2 gene mutations.

Missense mutations such as R279W cause an amino acid substitution (arginine to tryptophan), which alters but does not abolish the sulfate transporter activity. This is a recurrent mutation found in the Finnish population as well as in other Europeans; at the homozygous state, it results in *recessive multiple epiphyseal dysplasia* (*rMED*, OMIM #226900) with mildly shortened or normal stature. Exact data about its prevalence are not available. An example of "intermediate" mutation is IVS1+2T>C, a splicing mutation which in homozygosity leads to reduced levels of mRNA and related product. It is common in the Finnish population, probably because of a founder effect, but it has been found in Central Europe too. Homozygous individuals have an intermediate clinical phenotype, *diastrophic dysplasia* (*DTD*, OMIM #222600), associated with short stature (adult height 135–150 cm for males; 100–120 cm for females), joint contractures, and other characteristic clinical signs. Finally, mutations that produce null alleles, such as the above-cited R178X, lead to no detectable DTDST protein activity within chondrocytes, and in homozygous individuals result in an extremely severe skeletal dysplasia, achondrogenesis type 1B (*ACG1B*, OMIM #600972). This condition is characterized by extremely short limbs, severe hypodysplasia of the spine and the rib cage, and is invariably lethal [28]. No data on the prevalence of ACG1B are available.

3. Bone disorders featuring short stature: osteogenesis imperfecta

Osteogenesis imperfecta (*OI*) is a chondro-osseous dysplasia characterized by fragile, deformed bones, short stature, and low bone mass (incidence: 1:15–20,000 births). Traditionally, it has been considered a bone disorder due to defects in type I collagen, the most abundant protein of bone, skin, and tendon extracellular matrices. In fact, 85–90% of OI cases are caused by dominant mutations in either of two genes, COL1A1 and COL1A2, causing both quantitative and structural defects in collagen [29]. Within the past decade, the discovery of new disease genes has exceeded the idea of OI as a collagen-related disorder. Recessively inherited forms of OI with lethal to moderately severe phenotypes may be caused by defects in genes whose products are involved in post-translational modifications and/or folding of type I collagen [30–32]. Finally, recent molecular findings of causative mutations for both dominant and recessive forms of OI in non-collagenous genes have enlightened new perspectives [33]. OI at present appears as a molecularly and phenotypically heterogenous disorder characterized by defective bone mineralization; moreover, since the recessive types of OI are caused by deficiency of proteins found in both cartilage and bone, a new concept of OI as chondro-osseous dysplasia is arising. The classification has evolved with the new genetic discoveries. The original classification of Sillence *et al.* (1979), divided OI in four types, from mild to lethal, on the basis of clinical and radiographic features [34]. **Table 1** summarizes an updated classification of different OI forms along with their causative genes and their effect on growth deficiency. The disease genes list will almost certainly become longer with time, thanks to the whole exome new sequencing approaches. From the biologist's perspective, a logical and "user-friendly" classification pools the genetic types on the basis of altered intracellular or extracellular metabolic pathways.

3.1. Defects in collagen

Type I collagen is a heterotrimer made of two $\alpha 1$(I) and one $\alpha 2$(I) chains. It is synthesized as a procollagen molecule, with N-terminal and C-terminal globular domains flanking the helical domain. N-terminal and C-terminal propeptides are removed after secretion by specific proteases in the extracellular matrix. After processing, the collagen helices are capable of spontaneous assembly into fibrils, to be further stabilized by crosslinks. The helical domain is characterized by uninterrupted G-X-Y triplets since just the small glycine side chain fits the internal helical space. The most common genetic defects in dominant OI are missense mutations causing glycine substitutions within the helical domain and consequently structural defects in collagen heterotrimers. Gly substitutions delay helical folding and, in this way, promote post-translational overmodifications. Misfolded chains disturb intracellular metabolism, delay collagen secretion, and affect extracellular matrix deposition and mineralization. Phenotypic consequences vary depending on the nature of substituting amino acid, helical position, and chain type. In the $\alpha 1$(I) chain, substitutions with charged or branched side chains disrupt helix stability and are mostly lethal. In the $\alpha 2$(I) chain, substitutions are mainly non-lethal. Heterozygous COL1A1 loss-of-function mutations result in synthesis of reduced amount (about 50%) of structurally normal collagen and cause the mildest form of *OI* (*type I*). Heterozygous COL1A2 loss-of-function mutations in COL1A2 do not cause any apparent OI phenotype. Examples of COL1A1 and COL1A2 mutations and corresponding phenotypes are listed in **Table 2**.

3.2. Defects in collagen post-translational modifications

Procollagen undergoes several post-translational modifications, most of which occur in the endoplasmic reticulum. Such modifications are required for its correct folding, secretion, and extracellular matrix assembly. A complex of three proteins in a 1:1:1 ratio (CRTAP, P3H1, CyPB) called the 3-hydroxylation complex post-translationally modifies selected prolines in type I collagen chains in osteoblasts and type II collagen chains in chondrocytes. Deficiency of any of the three partners of the 3-hydroxylation complex, caused by loss-of-function mutations in both alleles of the corresponding gene, results in clinically distinct forms of moderate to lethal recessive OI (types VII, VIII, and IX, respectively, see **Table 1**). Common features are very low BMD, rhizomelia, bone fragility, and moderate to very severe growth deficiency. These recessive forms of OI are much rarer than the dominant forms (they account for 2–5% of OI cases detected in North America and Europe) and occur prevalently in inbred families.

Mode of Inheritance	OI type/ OMIM #	Defective gene	Defective protein	Cellular disturbance	Short stature*
Autosomal dominant (85–90% of OI cases)	I/#166200	COL1A1	Collagen I	Collagen quantitative defect	No
	II/#166210	COL1A1 or COL1A2	Collagen I	Collagen qualitative/ structural defect	Lethal
	III/#259420	COL1A1 or COL1A2	Collagen I	Qualitative/structural defect	+++
	IV/#166220	COL1A1 or COL1A2	Collagen I	Qualitative/structural defect	+
	V/#610967	IFITM5	BRIL	Bone matrix mineralization	+
Autosomal recessive (10–15% of OI cases)	VI/#613982	SERPINF1	PEDF	Bone matrix mineralization	++
	VII/#610682	CRTAP	CRTAP	Collagen hydroxylation	++
	VIII/#610915	LEPRE1	P3H1	Collagen hydroxylation	+++
	IX/#259440	PPIB	CyPB	Collagen hydroxylation	+/++
	X/#613848	SERPINH1	HSP47	Collagen chaperoning	+++
	XI/#610968	FKBP10	FKBP65	Collagen chaperoning	+
AR—very rare	XII/#613849	SP7/OX	OSTERIX	Osteoblast differentiation	+++
	XIII/#614856	BMP1	PICP endopeptidase	Abnormal procollagen I C-terminal propeptide processing	+++
	XIV/#615066	TMEM38B	TRIC-B	Intracellular [Ca modulation	+
	XV/#615220	WNT1	WNT1	Wnt signaling pathway (bone formation)	++
	XVI/#616229	CREB3L1	OASIS	Bone formation	+++

*+ = ~–1 SD; ++ = ~–2 SD; +++ = >–2 SD.

Table 1. OI types and related gene/protein defects.

OI type	Gene	Mutation	Phenotypic defect	Reference
I AD	COL1A1	c.757 C>T p. R253 stop	Haploinsufficiency (decreased amount of structurally normal collagen)	[35]
II AD	COL1A2	c.1874 G>A p.G625 D	Structurally abnormal collagen chains	[35]
III AD	COL1A1	c.2461 G>A p.G821 S	Structurally abnormal collagen chains	[35]
IV AD	COL1A2	c.577 G>A p.G193 S	Structurally abnormal collagen chains	[35]
V AD	IFITM5	c.-14 C>T p. +MALQP	Functionally abnormal IFITM5 protein (gain of function)	[36]
VI AR	SERPINF1	c.423delG + c.423delG p.I142Sfs*9	Lack of PEDF protein	[37]
VII AR	CRTAP	(c.118_133del16insTACCC)+ (c. 118_133del16insTACCC) p.Q40Yfs*117	Severe impairment of prolyl 3-hydroxylation complex activity (collagen post translational modification)	[38]
XI AR	FKBP10	c.1399+1G>A + c.1399+1G>A aberrant splicing	Lack of FKBP65 protein	[32]

Table 2. Examples of causative mutations in different types of OI found at the Verona molecular diagnostic center.

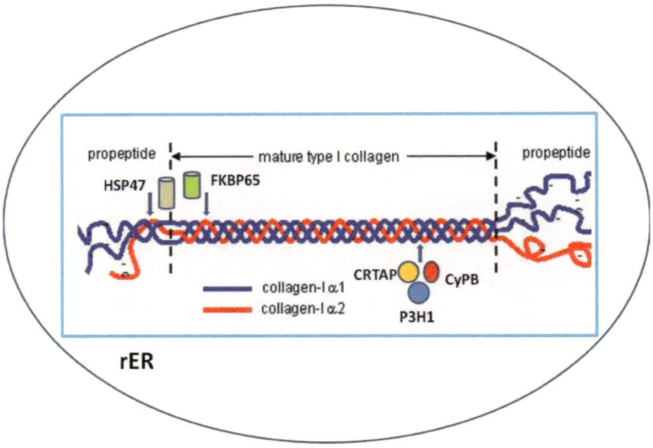

Figure 6. Type I collagen chains synthesis, post-translational modification and folding. Schematic representation of rough endoplasmic reticulum (rER) within an osteoblast. Several rER resident enzymes perform post-translational modifications on alpha 1 (blue) and alpha 2 (red) chains, before and during their folding. In particular, the prolyl 3-hydroxylation complex (P3H1 + CyPB + CRTAP) is shown. FKBP65 and HSP47 proteins are involved in subsequent maturation steps, such as folding and cross-linking, before secretion occurs. Defects, due to mutations in the corresponding genes, in any of the proteins shown in the figure, are responsible for several types of osteogenesis imperfecta (see text for details).

3.3. Defects in collagen folding and secretion

Folding of post-translationally modified α chains is assisted by ER-resident collagen-specific chaperones. Absence or dysfunction of two collagen chaperones, HSP47 and FKBP65, due to mutations in both alleles of the corresponding genes (SERPINH1 and FKBP10, respectively) have been reported to cause very rare recessive OI. A single patient has been reported so far with HSP47 deficiency and a severe *OI* phenotype (*type X*) with considerable growth deficiency [39]. Several patients with a milder form of *OI* (*type XI*) due to FKBP65 dysfunction have been reported, showing long bone fractures, short stature, and ligamentous laxity [40]. Common cellular features in these two clinically distinct forms are intracellular aggregation and delayed secretion of collagen, normally post-translationally modified, but unstable (increased sensitivity to protease digestion was demonstrated *in vitro*). These observations corroborate the idea that specific chaperones are necessary to monitor collagen helix folding and stabilization during transit through the secretory pathway. **Figure 6** schematically illustrates the role of gene products mentioned in Steps 3.1, 3.2, and 3.3.

3.4. Defects in bone mineralization

Autosomal-dominant *type V OI* and autosomal-recessive *type VI OI* were first described as distinctive forms of brittle bone disorder in 2000 and 2002, respectively, by Glorieux *et al.* on the basis of peculiar histological features revealing defects in the mineralization process [41, 42]. All patients with type V OI have distinctive mesh-like lamellation on bone histology; an osteoporotic phenotype associates paradoxically with exuberant bone formation in hypertrophic callus, affecting periosteal bone. As it was discovered in 2012, all

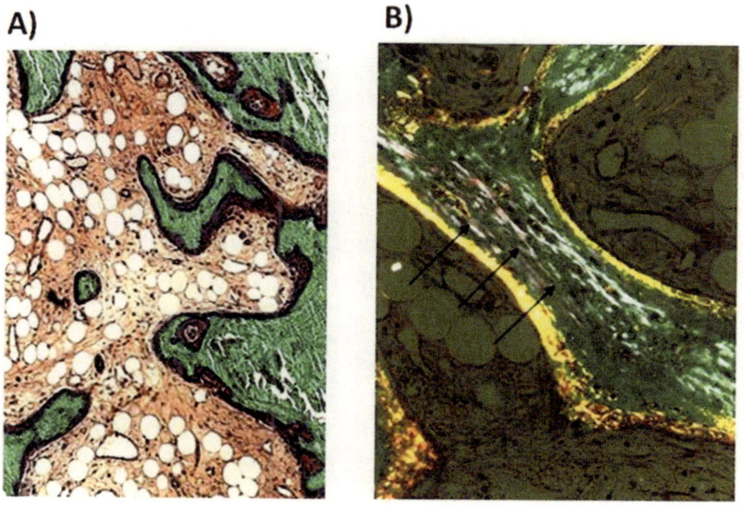

Figure 7. Defects in bone mineralization in OI type VI. (A) Goldner-stained iliac bone section of a OI type VI patient. Resorption lacunae and a large quantity of unmineralized osteoid (in red) are visible. (B) Bone section under polarized light. Arrows point to anomalies in the orientation of lamellae, reminiscent of a "fish-scale" pattern (magnification 200×). (Reproduced from J Bone Miner Res 2012; 50: 343–9 with permission of the American Society for Bone and Mineral Research).

patients with type V OI share the same heterozygous mutation (c.-14C>T) in the 5′UTR (untranslated transcribed region) of IFITM5 gene [43]. The mutation creates a novel start codon, thus adding five amino acids to the N-terminus of the protein, named BRIL, with a gain-of-function effect. BRIL is a transmembrane protein highly expressed in osteoblasts during mineralization. In the case of type VI OI, the causative gene is SERPINF1, which encodes for PEDF, a ubiquitously expressed multifunctional secreted protein. Patients affected by type VI OI, as well as the murine knockout model, do not produce PEDF because of different loss-of-function mutations in both SERPINF1 alleles [37, 44, 45]. Type VI OI children do not show skeletal abnormalities at birth, fractures do not occur until the age of 8–12 months, but a severe progressively deforming bone dysplasia with frequent long bone fractures develops thereafter. Various studies have demonstrated that PEDF, which is produced both by chondrocytes and osteoblasts, is necessary for osteoblast development, favoring the expression of osteogenic genes and mineral deposition. It stimulates the production of osteoprotegerin, thus inhibiting osteoclast maturation. The absence of PEDF is detrimental for bone homeostasis and osteoid mineralization. Type VI patients bone histology, in fact, reveals an increased amount of unmineralized osteoid and a peculiar fish-scale pattern under polarized light (**Figure 7**). Although mutations in IFITM5 and SERPINF1 seem to have opposite effects on mineralization-increased ectopic ossification in type V and reduced bone mineralization in type VI, further findings have demonstrated that the two gene products, BRIL and PEDF, do interplay in the process of bone mineralization [46].

3.5. Defects in osteoblast development

Mutations in two genes involved in osteoblast differentiation have been recently associated with recessive *OI* phenotypes: SP7 (*type XII*) and WNT1 (*type XV*). SP7 codes for a transcription regulator factor, OSTERIX, which plays an essential role in regulating the differentiation of preosteoblasts to osteoblasts. The unique type XII patient so far described [47], born to first-grade Egyptian cousins, harbors a homozygous frameshift mutation in SP7 gene which most likely leads to a dysfunctional OSTERIX protein. WNT1, a member of the Wnt family of secreted glycoproteins, is the activator of a complex intracellular signaling pathway. It plays an important role in bone formation and maintenance; the above-cited SP7 master gene and ALPL gene (which encode alkaline phosphatase, a key enzyme for bone mineralization) are among the downstream targets of Wnt signaling. Heterozygous WNT1 mutations may cause early-onset osteoporosis, while homozygous mutations impairing Wnt protein occur in patients with severe OI with short stature, frequent fractures, and vertebral compressions [48]. **Figure 8** illustrates schematically the role of gene products mentioned in Steps 3.4 and 3.5.

Schematic and simplified representation of the differentiation steps from bone marrow mesenchymal stem cell to mature osteoblast. The transcription factors with an inductive effect (RUNX2, OSTERIX) are indicated in red as well as the osteoblast-specific proteins PEDF and BRIL, as cited in the text. The WNT signaling pathway plays a crucial role in osteoblast differentiation, proliferation, and bone matrix formation/mineralization. Defects, due to

http://dx.doi.org/10.5772/64560

mutations in the corresponding genes, in any of the proteins shown in the figure, are responsible for various types of osteogenesis imperfecta (see the text for details).

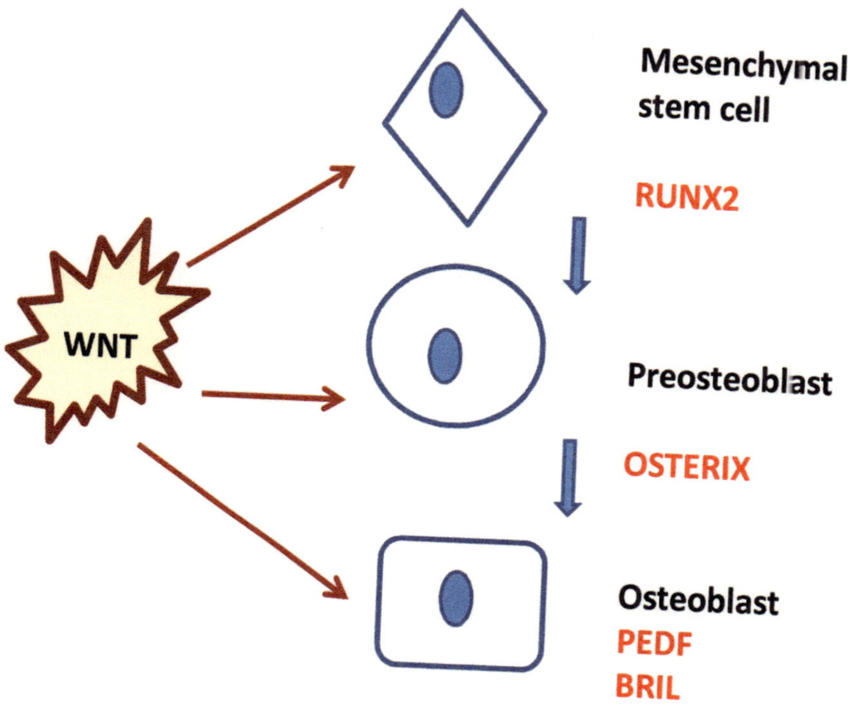

Figure 8. Osteoblast development.

3.6. Restricted growth in OI

Short stature is the most prevalent secondary feature of OI [49]. Only in the mildest form, OI type I, affected individuals have minimal bone deformities and normal stature. In all other types of OI, mild/moderate (+/++) to very severe (+++) growth deficiency is to be found (see **Table 1**). Short stature in OI is not caused by premature closure of growth plates; it can be the consequence of compromised extracellular matrix structure and mineralization, which impact on bone properties, leading to repeated long bones fractures, deformities, and bowing. Severely affected patients may be short because of vertebral compression fractures, severe scoliosis, lower limb deformities, and disruption of growth plates. However, growth can also be delayed in the absence of these abnormalities. The mean standing height of patients with OI is lower than that of their unaffected first-degree family members, regardless of severity. Truncal height is reduced, and head size increased in one-third of the patients with moderate or severe OI.

During childhood, there appears to be no difference between the standing heights of girls and boys, but women have lower height *z*-scores than men. The reduction in arm span *z*-score generally follows the same pattern as for height: individuals with moderate or severe OI tend to have lower z-scores than individuals with mild OI. The arm span/height ratio appears to be increased in children with moderate or severe OI, but not in those with mild OI. Mean concentrations of insulin-like growth factor (IGF)-I and IGF-binding protein (IGFBP)-3 are generally normal, in the low range of age-specific reference values. Growth hormone (GH) deficiency is very rare in patients with OI [50]. The etiology of the growth restriction in children with moderate and severe OI is not entirely clear. It has been suggested that it could be viewed as a self-protective mechanism: a given mechanical load creates smaller stresses in a short bone than in a long bone; thus, a short bone will break less easily [51]. People with severe OI have a typical deformity of the growth cartilage, defined as "popcorn" appearance of the metaphysis. Microfractures of the growth cartilage may play a role in the growth problems experienced by these patients. There are no reports on the effects of puberty and hormonal changes on growth in children with OI.

3.7. Conclusions

The intent of this chapter was to give a molecular and cellular overview of selected conditions associated with impaired height, focusing on growth plate misregulation, cartilage extracellular matrix dysfunctions, osteoblast differentiation, and mineralization process impairments.

4. Methods

Most of the experimental data described in this chapter come from either *in vitro* studies performed on cultured cells or from *in vivo* studies performed on animal models.

4.1. *In vitro* cell cultures

Cell culture studies on mutated FGFR3 were mostly performed in chondrosarcoma RCS cells from rat, ATDC5 from mouse, or in heterologous cell lines as Hek293 or PC12. Single-codon substitutions were introduced into the cDNA encoding FGFR3 by site-directed mutagenesis, and the plasmids carrying different mutant molecules were transfected into cultured cells to allow protein expression. To address questions related to the biochemistry of mutant FGFR3 molecules, which is assessing the degree of receptor activation, FGFR3 proteins were isolated from cell lysates by immunoprecipitation techniques and analyzed by Western blot using specific antibodies directed to phosphorylated tyrosine. Intracellular receptor localization was visualized by immunofluorescence [22].

Studies in the field of O.I. are mostly based on cultivation of fibroblasts obtained (upon informed consent) from patients' skin biopsies. Fibroblasts are grown in DMEM medium supplemented with 10% fetal bovine serum (FBS), 2 mM L-glutamine, and antibiotics (penicillin and streptomycin) at standard concentration. Proteins, DNA, and mRNA are extracted and purified from cells for subsequent analyses. Detailed description of methods can be found in Refs [31, 38].

4.2. Animal models

Transgenic mice described in the chapter were generated by targeting the specific genes of interest in murine embryonic stem cells with the homologous recombination technique, originally described by Thomas AND Capecchi [52]. Several mouse models orthologous to human skeletal dysplasia have been generated where gene expression was targeted to chondrocytes. The list includes ACH, TDI, TDII, and SADDAN [53, 54]). Histochemical analyses were performed on tissues isolated from proximal tibial growth plate tissue, generally prepared from 1-week-old mice.

4.3. Gene sequencing

The search of causative mutations described in the text was performed by sequencing exons and exon/intron boundaries of the candidate genes. Typically, single exons are amplified by PCR using appropriate primers and then subjected to automated sequencing according to standard protocols. When analysis of known established disease genes failed to identify the causative mutations, whole exome sequencing strategies were employed in order to identify novel loci [55, 56].

4.4. Growth plate histology

For analyses on human samples, tibial and/or femoral cartilage fragments were obtained from medically aborted fetuses upon informed parental consent. Pregnancies were legally terminated after ultrasonographic and X-ray detection of severe dwarfism.

4.5. Bone histology

Biopsies obtained from iliac crest (upon informed consent) are fixed in 70% ethanol and embedded undecalcified in methylmethacrylate resin. Bone sections are cut by microtome, stained by Goldner's stain, and mounted on microscope slides.

Acknowledgements

We thank Mr Gabriele Liboi for his skilful contribution to **Figure 1**.

Author details

Monica Mottes* and Patricia Marie-Jeanne Lievens

*Address all correspondence to: monica.mottes@univr.it

Section of Biology and Genetics, Department of Neurosciences, Biomedicine and Movement Sciences, University of Verona, Verona, Italy

References

[1] Durand C, Rappold GA. Height matters – from monogenic disorders to normal variation. Nat Rev Endocrinol. 2013;9(3):171–7. doi: 10.1038/nrendo.2012.251

[2] Rimoin DL. The chondrodystrophies. Adv Hum Genet. 1975;5:1–118.

[3] Horton WA, Degnin CR. FGF in endochondral skeletal development. Trends Endocrinol Metab. 2009;20(7):341–8. doi: 10.1016/j.tem.2009.04.003. Epub 2009 Aug 27.

[4] Foldynova-Trantirkova S, Wilcox WR, Krejci P. Sixteen years and counting: the current understanding of fibroblast growth factor receptor 3 (FGFR3) signaling in skeletal dysplasias. Hum Mutat. 2012;33(1):29–41. doi: 10.1002/humu.21636. Epub 2011 Nov 16.

[5] Ornitz DM, Marie PJ. Fibroblast growth factor signaling in skeletal development and disease. Genes Dev. 2015;29(14):1463–86. doi: 10.1101/gad.266551.115

[6] Colvin JS, Bohne BA, Harding GW, McEwen DG, Ornitz DM. Skeletal overgrowth and deafness in mice lacking fibroblast growth factor receptor 3. Nat Genet. 1996;12(4): 390–7.

[7] Toydemir RM, Brassington AE, Bayrak-Toydemir P, Krakowiak PA, Jorde LB, Whitby FG, Longo N, Viskochil DH, Carey JC, Bamshad MJ. A novel mutation in FGFR3 causes camptodactyly, tall stature, and hearing loss (CATSHL) syndrome. Am J Hum Genet. 2006;79(5):935–41. Epub 2006 Sep 26.

[8] Laederich MB, Horton WA. FGFR3 targeting strategies for achondroplasia. Expert Rev Mol Med. 2012;14:e11. doi: 10.1017/erm.2012.4

[9] Shinde DN, Elmer DP, Calabrese P, Boulanger J, Arnheim N, Tiemann-Boege I. New evidence for positive selection helps explain the paternal age effect observed in achondroplasia. Hum Mol Genet. 2013;22(20):4117–26. doi: 10.1093/hmg/ddt260. Epub 2013 Jun 4.

[10] Wang Y, Spatz MK, Kannan K, Hayk H, Avivi A, Gorivodsky M, Pines M, Yayon A, Lonai P, Givol D. A mouse model for achondroplasia produced by targeting fibroblast factor receptor 3. Proc Natl Acad Sci U S A. 1999;96(8):4455–60.

[11] Monsonego-Ornan E, Adar R, Feferman T, Segev O, Yayon A. The transmembrane mutation G380R in fibroblast growth factor receptor 3 uncouples ligand-mediated receptor activation from down-regulation. Mol Cell Biol. 2000;20(2):516–22.

[12] Garofalo S, Kliger-Spatz M, Cooke JL, Wolstin O, Lunstrum GP, Moshkovitz SM, Horton WA, Yayon A. Skeletal dysplasia and defective chondrocyte differentiation by targeted overexpression of fibroblast growth factor 9 in transgenic mice. J Bone Miner Res. 1999;14(11):1909–15.

[13] Murakami S, Balmes G, McKinney S, Zhang Z, Givol D, de Crombrugghe B. Constitutive activation of MEK1 in chondrocytes causes Stat1-independent achondroplasia-like

dwarfism and rescues the Fgfr3-deficient mouse phenotype. Genes Dev. 2004;18(3): 290–305.

[14] Webster MK, Donoghue DJ. Constitutive activation of fibroblast growth factor receptor 3 by the transmembrane domain point mutation found in achondroplasia. EMBO J. 1996;15(3):520–7.

[15] Klag KA, Horton WA. Advances in treatment of achondroplasia and osteoarthritis. Hum Mol Genet, 2016, 25(R1):R2–R8.doi:10.1093/hmg/ddv419

[16] McKusick VA, Kelly TE, Dorst JP. Observations suggesting allelism of the achondroplasia and hypochondroplasia genes. J Med Genet. 1973;10(1):11–6.

[17] Bellus GA, McIntosh I, Smith EA, Aylsworth AS, Kaitila I, Horton WA, Greenhaw GA, Hecht JT, Francomano CA. A recurrent mutation in the tyrosine kinase domain of fibroblast growth factor receptor 3 causes hypochondroplasia. Nat Genet. 1995;10(3): 357–9.

[18] Tavormina PL, Shiang R, Thompson LM, Zhu YZ, Wilkin DJ, Lachman RS, Wilcox WR, Rimoin DL, Cohn DH, Wasmuth JJ. Thanatophoric dysplasia (types I and II) caused by distinct mutations in fibroblast growth factor receptor 3. Nat Genet. 1995;9(3):321–8.

[19] Lievens PM, Liboi E. The thanatophoric dysplasia type II mutation hampers complete maturation of fibroblast growth receptor 3 (FGFR3), which activates signal transducer and activator of transcription 1 (STAT1) from the endoplasmic reticulum. J Biol Chem. 2003;278(19):17344–9. Epub 2003 Mar 6.

[20] Lievens PM, Mutinelli C, Baynes D, Liboi E. The kinase activity of the fibroblast growth factor receptor 3 with activation loop mutations affects receptor trafficking and signaling. J Biol Chem. 2004;279(41):43254–60. Epub 2004 Aug 2.

[21] Tavormina PL, Bellus GA, Webster MK, Bamshad MJ, Fraley AE, McIntosh I, Szabo J, Jiang W, Jabs EW, Wilcox WR, Wasmuth JJ, Donoghue DJ, Thompson LM, Francomano CA. A novel skeletal dysplasia with developmental delay and acanthosis nigricans is caused by a Lys650Met mutation in the fibroblast growth factor receptor 3 gene. Am J Hum Genet. 1999;64(3):722–31.

[22] Lievens PM, Roncador A, Liboi E. K644E/M FGFR3 mutants activate Erk1/2 from the endoplasmic reticulum through FRS2 alpha and PLC gamma-independent pathways. J Mol Biol. 2006;357(3):783–92. Epub 2006 Feb 3.

[23] Posey KL, Alcorn JL, Hecht JT. Pseudoachondroplasia/COMP – translating from the bench to the bedside. Matrix Biol. 2014;37:167–73. doi: 10.1016/j.matbio.2014.05.006

[24] Hecht JT, Montufar-Solis D, Decker G, Lawler J, Daniels K, Duke PJ. Retention of cartilage oligomeric matrix protein (COMP) and cell death in redifferentiated pseudoachondroplasia chondrocytes. Matrix Biol. 1998;17(8–9):625–33.

[25] Svensson L, Aszódi A, Heinegård D, Hunziker EB, Reinholt FP, Fässler R, Oldberg A. Cartilage oligomeric matrix protein-deficient mice have normal skeletal development. Mol Cell Biol. 2002;22(12):4366–71.

[26] Satoh H, Susaki M, Shukunami C, Iyama K, Negoro T, Hiraki Y. Functional analysis of diastrophic dysplasia sulfate transporter. Its involvement in growth regulation of chondrocytes mediated by sulfate proteoglycans. J Biol Chem. 1998;273(20):12307–15.

[27] Rossi A, Superti-Furga A. Mutations in the diastrophic dysplasia sulfate transporter (DTDST) gene (SLC26A2): 22 novel mutations, mutation review, associated skeletal phenotypes, and diagnostic relevance. Hum Mutat. 2001;17(3):159–71.

[28] Superti-Furga A, Hastbacka J, Wilcox WR, Cohn DH, van der Harten HJ, Rossi A, et al. Achondrogenesis type IB is caused by mutations in the diastrophic dysplasia sulphate transporter gene. Nat Genet. 1996;12(1):100–2.

[29] Marini JC, Forlino A, Cabral WA, Barnes AM, San Antonio JD, Milgrom S, et al. Consortium for osteogenesis imperfecta mutations in the helical domain of type I collagen: regions rich in lethal mutations align with collagen binding sites for integrins and proteoglycans. Hum Mutat. 2007;28(3):209–21.

[30] Morello R, Bertin TK, Chen Y, Hicks J, Tonachini L, Monticone M, et al. CRTAP is required for prolyl 3-hydroxylation and mutations cause recessive osteogenesis imperfecta. Cell. 2006;127(2):291–304.

[31] Cabral WA, Chang W, Barnes AM, Weis M, Scott MA, Leikin S, et al. Prolyl 3-hydroxylase 1 deficiency causes a recessive metabolic bone disorder resembling lethal/severe osteogenesis imperfecta. Nat Genet. 2007;39(3):359–65. Erratum in: Nat Genet. 2008;40(7):927.

[32] Venturi G, Monti E, Dalle Carbonare L, Corradi M, Gandini A, Valenti MT, et al. A novel splicing mutation in FKBP10 causing osteogenesis imperfecta with a possible mineralization defect. Bone. 2012;50(1):343–9. doi: 10.1016/j.bone.2011.10.023

[33] Marini JC, Reich A, Smith SM. Osteogenesis imperfecta due to mutations in non-collagenous genes: lessons in the biology of bone formation. Curr Opin Pediatr. 2014;26(4):500–7. doi: 10.1097/MOP.0000000000000117

[34] Sillence DO, Senn A, Danks DM. Genetic heterogeneity in osteogenesis imperfecta. J Med Genet. 1979;16(2):101–16.

[35] Venturi G,Tedeschi E, Mottes M, Valli M, Camilot M, Viglio S, Antoniazzi F, Tatò L. Osteogenesis imperfecta: clinical, biochemical and molecular findings. Clin Genet. 2006 Aug;70(2):131–9. Erratum in Clin Genet. 2006 Nov;70(5):455.

[36] Corradi M, Monti E, Venturi G, Gandini A, Mottes M, Antoniazzi F. The recurrent causal mutation for osteogenesis imperfecta type V occurs at a highly methylated CpG dinucleotide within the IFITM5 gene. Journal of Pediatric Genetics 3 (2014) 35–39 DOI 10.3233/PGE-14079

[37] Venturi G, Gandini A, Monti E, Dalle Carbonare L, Corradi M, Vincenzi M, et al. Lack of expression of SERPINF1, the gene coding for pigment epithelium-derived factor, causes progressively deforming osteogenesis imperfecta with normal type I collagen. J Bone Miner Res. 2012;27(3):723–8. doi: 10.1002/jbmr.1480

[38] Valli M, Barnes AM, Gallanti A, Cabral WA, Viglio S, Weis MA, et al. Deficiency of CRTAP in non-lethal recessive osteogenesis imperfect reduces collagen deposition into matrix. Clin Genet. 2012;82(5):453–9. doi 10.1111/j.1399-0004.2011.01794

[39] Christiansen HE, Schwarze U, Pyott SM, AlSwaid A, Al Balwi M, Alrasheed S, et al. Homozygosity for a missense mutation in SERPINH1, which encodes the collagen chaperone protein HSP47, results in severe recessive osteogenesis imperfecta. Am J Hum Genet. 2010;86(3):389–98. doi: 10.1016/j.ajhg.2010.01.034

[40] Alanay Y, Avaygan H, Camacho N, Utine GE, Boduroglu K, Aktas D, et al. Mutations in the gene encoding the RER protein FKBP65 cause autosomal-recessive osteogenesis imperfecta. Am J Hum Genet. 2010;86(4):551–9. doi: 10.1016/j.ajhg.2010.02.022

[41] Glorieux FH, Rauch F, Plotkin H, Ward L, Travers R, Roughley P, et al. Type V osteogenesis imperfecta: a new form of brittle bone disease. J Bone Miner Res. 2000;15(9): 1650–8.

[42] Glorieux FH, Ward LM, Rauch F, Lalic L, Roughley PJ, Travers R. Osteogenesis imperfecta type VI: a form of brittle bone disease with a mineralization defect. J Bone Miner Res. 2002;17(1):30–8.

[43] Cho TJ, Lee KE, Lee SK, Song SJ, Kim KJ, Jeon D, et al. A single recurrent mutation in the 5'-UTR of IFITM5 causes osteogenesis imperfecta type V. Am J Hum Genet. 2012;91(2):343–8. doi: 10.1016/j.ajhg.2012.06.005

[44] Homan EP, Rauch F, Grafe I, Lietman C, Doll JA, Dawson B, et al. Mutations in SERPINF1 cause osteogenesis imperfecta type VI. J Bone Miner Res. 2011;26(12):2798–803. doi: 10.1002/jbmr.487

[45] Bogan R, Riddle RC, Li Z, Kumar S, Nandal A, Faugere MC, et al. A mouse model for human osteogenesis imperfecta type VI. J Bone Miner Res. 2013;28(7):1531–6. doi: 10.1002/jbmr.1892

[46] Farber CR, Reich A, Barnes AM, Becerra P, Rauch F, Cabral WA, et al. A novel IFITM5 mutation in severe atypical osteogenesis imperfecta type VI impairs osteoblast production of pigment epithelium-derived factor. J Bone Miner Res. 2014;29(6):1402–11.

[47] Lapunzina P, Aglan M, Temtamy S, Caparrós-Martín JA, Valencia M, Letón R, et al. Identification of a frameshift mutation in Osterix in a patient with recessive osteogenesis imperfecta. Am J Hum Genet. 2010;87(1):110–4. doi: 10.1016/j.ajhg.2010.05.016

[48] Laine CM, Joeng KS, Campeau PM, Kiviranta R, Tarkkonen K, Grover M, et al. WNT1 mutations in early onset osteoporosis and osteogenesis imperfecta. N Engl J Med. 2013;368(19):1809–16. doi: 10.1056/NEJMoa1215458

[49] Plotkin H. Growth in osteogenesis imperfecta. GGH J. 2007;23(2):17–23. Available from: www.GGHjournal.com

[50] Marini JC, Bordenick S, Heavner G, Rose S, Hintz R, Rosenfeld R, Chrousos GP. The growth hormone and somatomedin axis in short children with osteogenesis imperfecta. J Clin Endocrinol Metab. 1993;76(1):251–6.

[51] Zeitlin L, Rauch F, Plotkin H, Glorieux FH. Height and weight development during four years of therapy with cyclical intravenous pamidronate in children and adolescents with osteogenesis imperfecta types I, III, and IV. Pediatrics. 2003;111(5 Pt 1):1030–6.

[52] Thomas KR, Capecchi MR. Site-directed mutagenesis by gene targeting in mouse embryo-derived stem cells. Cell. 1987;51(3):503–12.

[53] Brodie SG, Deng CX. Mouse models orthologous to FGFR3-related skeletal dysplasia. Pediatr Pathol Mol Med. 2003;22(1):87–103.

[54] Iwata T, Li CL, Deng CX, Francomano CA. Highly activated Fgfr3 with the K644M mutation causes prolonged survival in severe dwarf mice. Hum Mol Genet. 2001;10(12): 1255–64.

[55] Becker J, Semler O, Gilissen C, Li Y, Bolz HJ, Giunta C, et al. Exome sequencing identifies truncating mutations in human SERPINF1 in autosomal-recessive osteogenesis imperfecta. Am J Hum Genet. 2011;88(3):362–71. doi: 10.1016/j.ajhg.2011.01.015

[56] Shaheen R, Alazami AM, Alshammari MJ, Faqeih E, Alhashmi N, Mousa N, et al. Study of autosomal recessive osteogenesis imperfecta in Arabia reveals a novel locus defined by TMEM38B mutation. J Med Genet. 2012;49(10):630–5. doi: 10.1136/jmedgenet-2012-101142

Chapter 5

Growth Hormone Receptor Signaling Pathways and its Negative Regulation by SOCS2

Leandro Fernández-Pérez, Amilcar Flores-Morales,
Borja Guerra, Juan C. Díaz-Chico and
Diego Iglesias-Gato

Additional information is available at the end of the chapter

http://dx.doi.org/10.5772/64606

Abstract

Growth hormone (GH) is a critical regulator of linear body growth during childhood but continues to have important metabolic actions throughout life. The GH receptor (GHR) is ubiquitously expressed, and deficiency of GHR signaling causes a dramatic impact on normal physiology during somatic development, adulthood, and aging. GHR belongs to a family of receptors without intrinsic kinase activity. However, GH binding to homodimers of GHR results in a conformational change in the receptors and the associated tyrosine kinase Janus kinase 2 (JAK2) molecules. Activated JAK2 phosphorylates the GHR cytoplasmic domain on tyrosine residues, and subsequent JAK2-dependent and JAK2-independent intracellular signal transduction pathways evoke cell responses including changes in gene transcription, proliferation, cytoskeletal reorganization, and lipid and glucose metabolism. JAK2 phosphorylates STAT5b, which is a key transcription factor in GH regulation of target genes associated with body growth, intermediate metabolism, and gender dimorphism; although STAT1, 3, and 5a have also been shown to be recruited by the GHR. In addition, many transcripts are regulated independently of STAT5b as a result of GHR activation of Src, ERK, and PI3K-mTOR signaling pathways. The analysis of molecular mechanisms involved in inactivation of GHR-dependent signaling pathway is also imperative for understanding GH physiology. This is clearly illustrated in the case of hepatic GHR-JAK2-STAT5b activation where signal duration regulates gender differences in liver gene expression. An early step in the termination of GH-dependent signaling is removal of GHRs by endocytosis and ubiquitination. The level of ubiquitin ligase SOCS2 is constitutively low, but its expression is rapidly induced by GH. SOCS2 binding to GHR complex promotes their ubiquitination and subsequent proteasomal degradation, contributing to the termination of the GH intracellular signaling. Clinically relevant, SOCS2 is a key negative regulator of GH-dependent body growth and lipid and glucose homeostasis. Furthermore, several cytokines, growth factors, xenobiotics, and sex hormones can regulate

SOCS2 protein level, which provides a mechanism for cross-talking where multiple factors can regulate GHR signaling during somatic development. A better understanding of this complex regulation in physiological and pathological states will contribute to prevent health damage and improve clinical management of patients with growth and metabolic disorders.

Keywords: GHR, SOCS2, Growth, Metabolism, sexual dimorphism

1. Introduction

Growth hormone (GH) is the main regulator of somatic growth through pleiotropic actions on systemic metabolism and local actions on the bone growth plate [1–4]. GH is predominantly linked to linear growth during childhood but continues to have important metabolic actions throughout life. Secreted from the pituitary gland, GH binds to its receptor (GHR) on the surface of the cells of the target tissues triggering a rapid cascade of intracellular signaling events, which leads to the expression of GH-regulated genes. This set of genes includes positive regulators of GH actions such as the one coding for the growth factor IGF-I, and also genes involved in the negative feedback mechanism responsible for the termination of the GHR intracellular signal, such as the suppressor of cytokine signaling 2 (SOCS2). In this chapter, we will review the current knowledge about the intracellular GH signaling as well as the role of SOCS2 in this regulation and discuss the implications on body growth.

2. Intracellular GH signaling

GH exerts its intracellular actions via the GHR that is ubiquitously expressed (e.g., liver, fat, muscle, bone, and lymphocytes). The GHR belongs to a family of transmembrane cytokine receptors that lack intrinsic enzymatic activity [5]. Instead, in order to activate intracellular signaling, the GHR cytosolic domain associates to the tyrosine kinase Janus kinase 2 (JAK2) [5]. Upon binding, GH promotes the dimerization of two GHR proteins, which results in a conformational change that triggers the activation of the associated tyrosine kinase JAK2 due to the unmasking of their kinase domain [5]. JAK2 activation triggers cross-phosphorylation event on the two adjacent JAK2 proteins and the phosphorylation of tyrosine residues on the cytosolic domain of the GHR. Signal transducer and activator of transcription (STAT) proteins are then recruited to these phosphorylated tyrosines (pY), where they themselves become substrates of JAK2. Although STAT1, STAT3, and STAT5a can also be recruited to the GHR, STAT5b is the main mediator of GH signaling [1, 3, 6]. Phosphorylation by JAK2 releases STAT5b from the receptor and promotes the formation of STAT5b dimer complexes. STAT5b homodimers translocate to the nucleus, bind to their response elements (TTCNNNGAA) on the DNA, and regulate the transcription of GH target genes (e.g., IGF-1, SOCS2, CYP2C12, and HNF6 [7–10]). Studies of human subjects carrying rare inactivation mutations in the GHR, STAT5b, and IGF-I genes have demonstrated the essentiality of this pathway for normal human growth. Individuals carrying these mutations exhibit severe dwarfisms with very similar growth curves [11–15]. Although STAT proteins are critical for many actions of GH [6], GH activation of JAK2 can initiate signaling pathways in addition to the STAT transcription factors as a result of GHR activation of: (1) the MAPK (Mitogen Activated Protein Kinase) pathway; (2) insulin receptor substrate (IRS) proteins implicated in the activation of the phosphatidylinositol-3-kinase (PI3K) and Akt pathway; (3) signal regulatory protein α (SIRPα), a transmembrane scaffold protein that recruits proteins including the tyrosine phosphatase SHP2; and (4) SH2B1, a scaffold protein that can activate JAK2 and enhance GH regulation of the actin cytoskeleton [6].

3. SOCS2 mediates GHR turnover

The analysis of molecular mechanisms involved in the inactivation of the GHR-dependent signaling pathway is also imperative for understanding GH physiology. This is clearly illustrated in the case of hepatic GHR-JAK2-STAT5b activation where signal duration regulates gender differences in liver gene expression [10]. Studies on primary hepatocytes and several cell lines have shown that GH-induced activation of JAK2-STAT5b is transient, with maximal activation achieved within the first 30 min of stimulation, followed by a period of inactivation. This period is characterized by an inability to achieve maximal JAK2-STAT5b activation by GH in the following 3–4 h, unless GH is withdrawn from the media [16]. Similarly, the male pattern of pituitary GH secretion in rats is episodic with peaks every 3–4 h with unmeasurable basal levels. Consequently, intracellular activation of STAT5b is also episodic and periods with low GH circulating levels are required to achieve maximal activation of STAT5b. On the other hand, female rats, which exhibit a more continuous GH secretion pattern with higher basal levels and smaller, irregular, and intermittent peaks, show reduced STAT5b activation compared with their males counterparts [17].

An early and important step in the termination of GH-dependent signaling is the removal of GHRs from the cell surface by mechanisms of endocytosis, which are dependent on ubiquitination [18]. SOCS2 is part of an E3 ubiquitin ligase complex with a key role in the negative regulation of GHR-JAK2-STAT5b signaling pathway, acting in a classical negative feedback loop manner [19–22]. The transcription of SOCS2 is induced by STAT5b in response to GH stimulation—which leads to elevated SOCS2 protein levels [16]—consistent with the critical role of STAT5b for growth [7] (**Figure 1**). SOCS2 binds to phosphorylated tyrosines at the GHR cytosolic domain through its SH2 domain while recruits Elongin B and C, the scaffold protein Cullin5, and the ring finger protein Rbx2 through its SOCS box domain to assemble an E3 ubiquitin ligase complex that ubiquitinates the GHR and promotes its internalization [23, 24] (**Figure 2**). These GHR-containing early endosomes are later fused to the lysosomes leading to GHR degradation [24]. In addition to SOCS2, the ubiquitin ligase β-TRCP has also been shown to mediate GHR ubiquitination and internalization with the key difference that this process is not GH dependent and the mechanism seems to act independently from SOCS2 [25]. Therefore, the current evidence would suggest that GHR membrane content is controlled by ubiquitin driven endocytosis [18]. The constitutive internalization of GHR is mediated by β-

TRCP, which is further enhanced upon GH induction of SOCS2 expression and function. Furthermore, the SH2 domain of SOCS2 can also bind to other components of the signaling cascade interfering with the propagation of the signal. Particularly, SOCS2 binds the GHR at Tyr487 and Tyr595 to prevent GHR signaling [21, 22]. The activation loop of JAK2 is also a target of SOCS2 that prevents JAK2 tyrosine phosphorylation and activation of STATs [16].

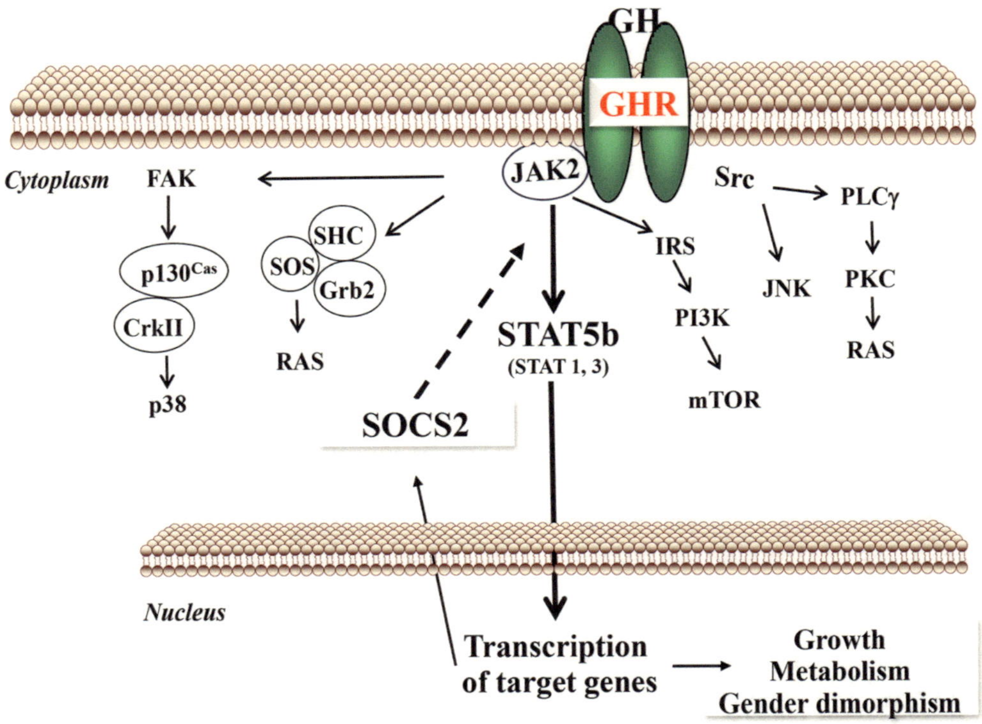

Figure 1. Negative regulation of GHR-STAT5b signaling pathway by SOCS2: The JAK2-STAT5b signal transduction pathway requires an exquisite cellular control and loss of its regulation can promote alterations in body growth. Intracellular activation of GHR-JAK2-STAT5b signaling pathway is transient and it is followed by a period of inactivation that is characterized by an inability to achieve maximal JAK2-STAT5b activation by GH. GHR-STAT5b activity induces the transcription of SOCS2 that acts as part of an E3 ubiquitin ligase complex that plays a key role in the negative regulation of GHR-JAK2-STAT5b signaling pathway.

The physiological role of SOCS2 as negative regulator of GH signaling was clearly demonstrated after the engineering of SOCS2-/- mice that are 40% larger than their wild-type (WT) mates. This phenotype of enlarged growth is not observed in mice lacking other members of the SOCS family such as SOCS1 or CIS (Cytokine-inducible SH2-containing protein), which strengthen the role of SOCS2 as key negative regulator of GH signaling. These *in vivo* studies highlight the role of SOCS2 as a key negative regulator of GH-dependent signaling and its role in the control of lipid and glucose homeostasis [26]. High SOCS2 expression levels have been found in the liver and the heart [16, 27], and, importantly, SOCS2 actions may not be confined to regulating GH signaling. There is evidence that SOCS2 can directly bind the IGF-IR, and,

http://dx.doi.org/10.5772/64606

therefore, it is possible that SOCS2 also regulates IGF-I signaling, although IGF-I does not induce SOCS2 expression [28, 29]. In addition, SOCS2 has been shown to inhibit signaling by IL-6, LIF, IGF-I, and prolactin (Prl) [19].

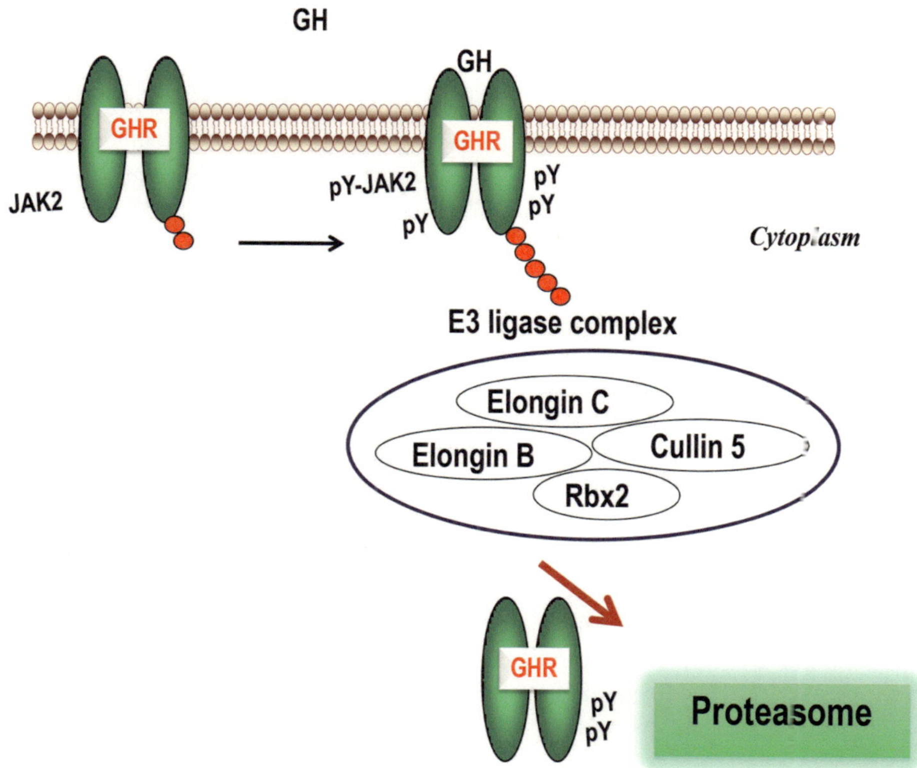

Figure 2. E3 ligase activity of SOCS2 and GHR degradation by proteasome: SOCS2 is part of an E3 ubiquitin ligase complex with a key role in the negative regulation of GHR-JAK2-STAT5b signaling pathway. SOCS2 binds to phosphorylated tyrosines (pY) at GHR cytosolic domain while recruits Elongin B and C, the scaffold protein Cullin5, and the ring finger protein Rbx2 to assemble an E3 ubiquitin ligase complex that mediates ubiquitination of target proteins (e.g., GHR) and their subsequent proteasomal degradation. The activation loop of JAK2 is also a target of SOCS2 that prevents JAK2 tyrosine phosphorylation and activation of STATs.

4. Other mechanisms of GHR signaling inhibition

In addition to SOCS2, GHR signaling induces the expression of other SOCS family members (SOCS-1, -3, and CIS) in a transient fashion. In vitro studies shown that SOCS1, SOCS3, and to a lesser extent CIS, are able to inhibit GHR signaling [30, 31]. Both SOCS1 and SOCS3 can directly bind phosphorylated JAK proteins via their SH2 domains inhibiting the kinase activity through the N-terminal kinase inhibitory region (KIR) [32]. Knockouts (-/-) of SOCS1 and SOCS3 genes are incompatible with life. SOCS1-/- mice died soon after birth due to hyperactivation of INFγ signaling. Combination of SOCS1 deletion with genetic depletion of INFγ or treatment with anti-INFγ antibodies ameliorates this phenotype [33]. Under these conditions, no changes in body growth have been reported, suggesting that SOCS1 may not play a major role in GHR signaling inhibition *in vivo*. On the other hand, CIS-/- mice exhibit no obvious phenotype, although overexpression of CIS results in restricted growth [16, 34]. Despite certain degree of redundancy within the SOCS family, the results obtained from mouse models suggest that SOCS2 is a major negative regulator of GH signaling *in vivo*. In addition to SOCS, the level of cell surface GHRs can be influenced by transcriptional, translational, and posttranslational factors (e.g., nutritional status, endocrine context, developmental stage, and sex steroids), which thereby regulate cell sensitivity to GH actions [16]. GHR translocation is also directly inhibited by IGF-I, likely contributing to a local feedback loop to hamper GH sensitivity [35]. As mutations in the GHR [15] and STAT5b genes [11] result in growth deficiencies, activating mutations of the tyrosine phosphatase SHP2 (PTPN11) also generates growth retardation linked to the Noonan syndrome [36]. PTPN11 is involved in the negative regulation of GH signaling, rendering lower IGF-I production after GH stimulation through regulation of the RAS/ERK1/2 pathway. Noonan syndrome driving PTPN11 mutants hyperactivates the RAS/ERK pathway in response to GH *in vitro* and *in vivo*, suggesting that GH-induced ERK1/2 activation could contribute to GHR signaling inactivation [36]. In the future, it will be interesting to study whether hyperactivation of ERK1/2 inhibit GHR through induction of SOCS expression [37]. Other protein phosphatases such as SHP1 and PTP1b (encoded by the PTPN6 and PTN1 genes, respectively) also play a role in controlling intracellular GH signaling. Upon GH stimulation, SHP1 translocates into the nucleus, where it binds to STAT5b inhibiting its activity [38]. SHP1 also interacts with phosphorylated JAK2 after GH stimulation, inhibiting the propagation of the signal, accordingly, SHP1-/- mice show prolonged GH signaling [39]. On the other hand, PTP1b is able to dephosphorylate GH-activated GHR and JAK2 [16, 40, 41].

5. GH regulation of body growth

Currently, it is accepted that GH is predominantly linked with postnatal growth, whereas IGF-I is linked with both pre and postnatal growth [42, 43]. The original somatomedin hypothesis, which proposed that pituitary GH increases tissue growth by stimulating production of hepatic IGF-I, has developed gradually, from a simple to a more complex form, by studies showing that (1) GH and IGF-I have both dual and overlapping functions on growth plate [44, 45]. However, there are still unanswered questions about the independent and combined relationships of GH and IGF-I on the growth plate and bone growth, including whether or not GH mediates any IGF-I independent effects on bone growth [46] and (2) conditional liver-specific IGF-I null mice exhibited body weights that were indistinguishable from wild-type littermates [47, 48]. These studies showed that, although the liver is the main source of circulating IGF-I, it is local IGF-I that is important for regulating postnatal growth [47]. Indeed, stimulation of hepatic IGF-I production in IGF-I null mice demonstrated that liver derived endocrine IGF-I contributes to 30% of adult body size and sustains postnatal development [49, 50]. In addition, GH is more effective than IGF-I because GH exerts additional growth-promoting actions independent of IGF-I. Previous studies have nicely demonstrated that STAT5b is important for sexual dimorphism of body growth (male-specific body growth) and liver gene expression [51]. Indeed, GH-dependent transcription of IGF-I is directly regulated by STAT5 [3], and the mode of GH administration (i.e., continuous vs. intermittent) influences GH actions on body growth rate, IGF-I expression, and STAT5b activity, which might be clinically relevant. Intermittent (male-like pattern) GH administration to rodents is a more potent stimulus of body growth rate, IGF-I expression, and STAT5b activity in liver than is continuous (female-like pattern) administration [17]. Global disruption of STAT5b in mice caused loss of sexually dimorphic growth characteristics, so that the affected males reduced their size to female size while female mice appeared unaffected. In addition, circulating IGF-I is reduced by 30–50% in affected male but not in female mice. In addition to STAT5b, other transcriptions factors are related with body growth. This is exemplified by the glucocorticoid receptor (GR), which is a critical coactivator of STAT5b in liver [52], or by interactions between estradiol (E2)/estrogen receptor alpha (ERα) signaling and STAT5 [53]. In addition to endocrine actions, paracrine involvement of STAT5a/b in the effects of GH on muscle is also evident in the loss of muscle IGF-I transcripts and mass seen with muscle-specific deletion of STAT5a/b [54].

6. SOCS2 and body growth

The importance of SOCS2 in the negative regulation of body growth through inhibition of GHR-JAK2-STAT5b signaling was further demonstrated using genetically modified mice. Thus, the SOCS2-/- overgrowth phenotype is fully dependent on GH and can be rescued by inhibiting GH expression in these mice by crossing them with Ghrhr$^{lit/lit}$ mice that have no circulating GH. Both the double-knockout mice and the Ghrhr$^{lit/lit}$ mice exhibited a similar 60% growth retardation. Furthermore, administration of GH to these knockout mice caused an increase of growth to a size indistinguishable from SOCS2-/- mice [21, 55]. Similarly, mice resulting from crossing SOCS2-/- with STAT5b-/- mice show growth rates close to wild-type mice [56]. Similar phenotypes to the SOCS2-/- mice have been observed in high-growth (hg) mice, a phenotype that occurs following spontaneous mutation in mouse chromosome 10 [57]. However, in contrast to SOCS2-/-, hg mice have higher plasma IGF-I levels [57]. Surprisingly, overexpression of SOCS2 results in a similar phenotype to SOCS2-/- mice [34, 58], which suggests that the effects of SOCS2 on GH signaling are dose-dependent, with dual effects [16, 58]. It has been proposed that at physiological levels, SOCS2 inhibits GH signaling, by promoting GHR degradation, but at higher doses, it inhibits signaling of other, more potent GH inhibiting SOCS (i.e., SOCS1 and 3) [34, 58]. This could be through association with SOCS3 binding sites on the GHR, thus blocking SOCS3 action, or by binding the other SOCS themselves and suppressing them through proteasomal degradation [22]. The validity of these mechanisms has been questioned [59] and their physiological relevance remains uncertain. A more likely explanation of the effects created by SOCS2 overexpression would be a disruption of its E3 ligase activity by sequestering components of the multimeric E3 ligase away from the GHR.

Several studies have demonstrated that polymorphisms in the GH/IGF-I/SOCS2 system can also modulate the efficacy of GH treatment in humans. In humans with GH insensitivity due to a GHR defects, growth retardation, and reduced bone density, which are the result of IGF-I deficiency, are observed [60]. More recently, abnormalities of STAT5b, the IGF-IR gene itself, and the binding proteins that influence IGF-I bioavailability at the tissue level have all been reported to be associated with a variable extent of short stature in humans [12]. The effects of GH treatment on growth can also be influenced by polymorphisms on GHR or IGFBP3 genes and by their interactions among polymorphisms [61–64]. Genetic polymorphisms in the SOCS2 gene have been associated with adult height variation in healthy individuals [13, 14, 65]. Recently, Braz et al. observed that SOCS2 polymorphism and its interaction with polymorphisms in GHR and IGFBP3 loci influenced the adult height of children with Turner syndrome and GHD (Growth Hormone Deficiency) after GH therapy [66]. Moreover, a SNP (Single Nucleotide Polymorphism) in the SOCS2 gene was reported associated to increased pubertal height in a Finnish cohort, supporting the role of SOCS2 in body growth in humans [67].

7. SOCS2 actions in bone and skeletal muscle

The overgrowth phenotype of the SOCS2 null (SOCS2-/-) mice [68] led to the confirmation that SOCS2 is a key effector of GH/IGF-I axis, in line with the anabolic role of GH on the skeleton [69, 70]. An interaction between SOCS2 and GH signaling in regulating body growth is consistent with the temporal increased expression of the GHR and the overgrowth of SOCS2-/- mice [68], with both occurring at around 3 weeks of age [68, 71]. Adult male SOCS2-/- mice are 40% heavier than their WT littermates while adult females reach the same size as the WT males [68]. Notably, the increased body weight of SOCS2-/- is not a result of any increase in fatty tissue but rather a proportional increase in size of most internal organs, muscle, and bone. SOCS2-/- mice have increased body length with longer longitudinal bones (femur, tibia, radius, and humerus) [68, 72]. No alterations to the growth plate were noted in the first description of SOCS2-/- mice [68]. Later investigations, however, found that epiphyseal chondrocytes express SOCS2 and growth plates from SOCS2-/- mice were enlarged with wider proliferative and hypertrophic zones. These findings were associated with an increased long bone length [72]. Recently, microtomography (μCT) analysis at 7 weeks of age showed that SOCS2-/- mice have increased bone mass (i.e., increased bone volume, trabecular number, and trabecular thickness), although these mice exhibit no difference in bone mineral density (BMD) compared to WT littermates [72]. In contrast, others authors have described lower trabecular and cortical bone mineral density in SOCS2-/- mice (at 4 and 15 weeks of age) as well as reduced cortical cross-sectional area and cortical thickness (at 4 weeks of age) [73]. Interestingly, these studies found elevated serum levels of osteocalcin (a marker of bone growth) [72, 73] and TRAP5 (a marker of osteoclast number) [72], which would indicate increased bone turnover in SOCS2-/- mice [68, 72]. Although circulating IGF-I levels are normal in SOCS2-/- mice [68, 72], they have elevated IGF-I mRNA in some tissues (heart, lung, and spleen but not liver, bone, fat, and muscle). Therefore, it is likely that the increased bone growth and observed structural differences within SOCS2-/- growth plates are a direct consequence of altered SOCS2-mediated

GH signaling at the growth plate [33, 72]. Recent studies of Dobie and coworkers support this hypothesis. Using *ex vivo* metatarsal cultures, they showed that GH was able to induce linear growth only in the absence of SOCS2 [74] via a mechanism that is independent of IGF-I.

In addition to increased bone length, enhanced GHR signaling by GH treatment or SOCS2 deficiency causes skeletal muscle enlargement [68]. The molecular effects of GH and SOCS2 on skeletal muscles are uncertain. GH actions on skeletal muscles are a consequence of its systemic metabolic effects but also in part mediated by hormone-induced changes in gene expression within the muscle, as demonstrated by studies that show GH-induced changes in gene expression, including SOCS2, in human [75, 76] and murine [77] skeletal muscles. SOCS2 also modulates signaling pathways in the muscle independently from GH. Using C2C12 mesenchymal precursor cells, Ouyang et al. have shown that SOCS2 interferes with myotube formation and favors the differentiation into osteoblast in a process that, although not fully understood, would require the regulation of JunB [78]. In line with these observations, SOCS2 would also suppress myotube formation by inhibiting mitochondria biogenesis by interfering with the p38/ATF2 pathway [79]. Overall, these investigations highlight the importance of SOCS2 actions on bone and muscle development and growth through the modulation of multiple pathways, not restricted to GH signaling. Moreover, SOCS2 plays a key role as mediator of the interplay between sex steroids and GH signaling in these tissues.

8. Other functions of GH in the regulation of body weight

Disruption of GHR-STAT5-SOCS2 signaling pathway is also associated with metabolic disorders [17, 26, 51, 80–84]. An inefficient GHR-JAK2-STAT5b signaling pathway results in fatty liver and adiposity in rodents and humans due to enhanced lipogenesis and reduced triglyceride secretion as well as reduced lipolysis [4, 80, 81]. This is supported by original findings showing that STAT5b null male mice become obese in later life [51] and that STAT5b deletion in a mature human was associated with obesity [85]. Therefore, GHR activated STAT5b plays a critical role in regulation of key enzymes involved in lipid and energy balance. Liver-specific GHR ablation leads to fatty liver because of reduced STAT5 activation despite normal plasma free fatty acid and minimal adiposity. Relevant to this review, agonists of liver X receptor (LXR), which cause hepatic steatosis [86], inhibit GH-STAT5b signaling [87]. This inhibition is mediated by SREBP1, a LXR target gene, through the downregulation of STAT5b gene transcription and stimulation of STAT5b protein degradation [87]. In contrast, ablation of SOCS2 in mice, which increased STAT5 signaling, protects them from high-fat diet-induced liver steatosis by increasing hepatic triglyceride secretion. As a result, these mice have increased peripheral fat accumulation both in adipose and muscle tissues. Although this is not associated with changes in systemic insulin sensitivity when mice are fed on a normal chow diet, under high-fat diet conditions, SOCS2-/- mice are glucose intolerant and insulin resistant and show increased expression of inflammatory cytokines [26]. The latter has been suggested to be a consequence of increased sensitivity of SOCS2-/- macrophages to lipopolysaccharide (LPS), leading to increased NF*k*B activation and inflammatory signaling in the liver despite reduced steatosis [26]. In contrast, SOCS2 deletion protected against streptozotocin-induced type I diabetes in adult male mice presumably by enhancing antiapoptotic actions of STAT5b [88]. Notably, SOCS2 can regulate inflammation by modulating the actions of other inflammatory cytokines [89]. The role of SOCS2 in the regulation of the inflammatory response seems to be independent of GH signaling. Furthermore, the effects of inflammatory cytokines on SOCS2 have been poorly investigated, with evidence that some interleukins induce SOCS2 gene expression only in specific cell types [89]. Thus, it has recently reported that in a sheep model, a point mutation in the SOCS2 gene not only resulted in higher body weight and size but also elevated leukocytes count in the milk as a sign of enhanced inflammatory response [90]. In addition, altered SOCS2 expression has also been associated with malignancies [84, 91–93]. Therefore, how to target SOCS2-regulated pathways without causing negative side effects that systemic and chronic reduction in SOCS2 protein might cause is still a challenge.

9. SOCS2 mediates the cross-talk between steroids and GH

Until recently, most studies concerning the interaction among GH and steroids have been focused on the influence of sex steroids on gender-specific pituitary GH secretion that has a great impact on hepatic transcriptional regulation [17, 94]. However, a direct target of steroids may also occur because interaction with androgen receptor (AR), estrogen receptor alpha or GR, and the signaling pathways linked to these receptors are connected with lipid and glucose homeostasis [95] and tissue growth [96, 97]. The relationship between GH and sex steroids relative to body growth has been extensively studied, but it is not fully understood. Sex steroids can directly modulate pituitary GH secretion [94, 98] in a process that in men seems to require prior aromatization of testosterone into estrogen [99] but also indirectly through regulating liver IGF-1 production. Thus, hypogonadal children have reduced GH secretion [100, 101] and girls with precocious puberty show increased levels [102]. Additionally, sex steroids also exert GH-independent effects on growth [103, 104]. During puberty, children experience a growth spurt concomitant with increasing levels of gonadal steroids and GH secretions [98, 103]. This pubertal growth spurt has been attributed primarily to the actions of estrogens [105], acting directly on the growth plate cartilage inducing proliferation and finally promoting epiphyseal fusion [106]. Thus, in girls with Turner syndrome, hormone replacement therapy results in growth spurt [107]. Due to these effects on bone maturation, pharmacological doses of sex steroids have been used in prepubertal children with the nonpathological condition of constitutionally tall stature to limit their final height since 1950s [108, 109].

At the molecular level, increasing amount of evidences suggests that SOCS2 as a key mediator of the interplay between GH and steroid hormones. Both androgens and estrogens are able to induce the expression of SOCS2, which in turn limits GH signaling in cells from different tissue origins such as liver, breast, and prostate [84, 110]. Transcriptional induction of SOCS2 expression by sex steroids is mediated by the steroid receptors, AR, for androgens, and ERα, in the case of estrogens. This activation seems to be mediated by STAT5 [84] in a similar fashion to what happened with another steroid receptor, the GR, which acts as cofactor for STAT5-mediated transcription of SOCS2 after glucocorticoid stimulation [27]. Thus, direct upregulation of SOCS2 expression by steroid hormones would limit GH actions on target tissues. The

http://dx.doi.org/10.5772/64606

liver, a major target tissue of GH, expresses both AR and ERα. Therefore, SOCS2 might play a central role in the modulation of GH signaling by androgens and estrogens which defines the gender dimorphism in response to GH. In good agreement to the role of SOCS2 as mediator of sex steroids and GH signaling, SOCS2 KO mice show a less pronounced growth reduction after E2 treatment than their WT mates (unpublished observations). Recently, Bolamperti and colleagues described a novel SOCS2 regulation by estradiol in human osteoblasts [111]. Here, E2 induces GH signaling (STAT5 phosphorylation after treatment with GH) by inhibiting SOCS2 expression through a mechanism that involves proteasomal degradation of the protein but not genomic actions. The molecular characterization of this regulation, e.g., whether these effects are ER mediated, as well as the elucidation of this regulation as a general mechanism or whether it is restricted to osteoblast cells deserve further investigation. Overall, steroids in general and sex steroids in particular can modulate GH actions by controlling SOCS2 expression in several ways and in a tissue-specific manner. In the liver, SOCS2 induction by steroids would modulate central metabolism as well as influence IGF-I secretion that in turn affects GH secretion. In the bone, however, estrogens would potentiate GH actions by reducing the expression of SOCS2.

10. General conclusions

GH is the main regulator of somatic growth through pleiotropic actions on systemic metabolism and local actions on the bone growth plate. Relevant is the critical role of SOCS2 for the negative regulation of body growth. However, many aspects on the actions of SOCS2 in physiological and pathological models have yet to be understood. Particularly, more studies investigating the mechanisms by which SOCS2 regulates metabolism (e.g., lipid metabolism), insulin actions, malignancies, or GHR signaling at the growth plate are certainly needed. Notably, how to target the elements of the SOCS2-regulated pathways without causing negative side effects that systemic and chronic reduction in SOCS2 protein might cause is still a challenge. Finally, the consequences of long-term exposition to steroid compounds (particularly, sex hormones-related compounds) on normal development, as a consequence of their influence on GHR signaling, are largely unknown. Understanding this complex interaction in physiological and pathological states could contribute to prevent health damage and improve clinical management of patients with somatic growth disorders.

Acknowledgements

We thank all the authors that have made a contribution to the understanding of the negative regulation of GHR signaling. We apologize to those whose work deserves to be cited but unfortunately are not quoted because of space limitations. The research program in the author's lab was supported by grants-in-aid from the Spanish Ministry of Economy and Competitiveness (MINECO) with the funding of European Regional Development Fund, European Social Fund, and Alfredo Martin-Reyes Foundation (Arehucas)—Canary Islands

Foundation for Cancer Research (FICIC). D.I.-G. and A.F.-M. are supported by grants from the Novo Nordisk Foundation and the Danish Cancer Society.

Author details

Leandro Fernández-Pérez[1*], Amilcar Flores-Morales[2,3], Borja Guerra[1], Juan C. Díaz-Chico[1] and Diego Iglesias-Gato[2,3]

*Address all correspondence to: leandrofco.fernandez@ulpgc.es

1 Institute for Research in Biomedicine and Health (IUIBS), University of Las Palmas de Gran Canaria (ULPGC), Molecular and Translational Pharmacology-BioPharm Group, Las Palmas, Spain

2 Faculty of Health Sciences, University of Copenhagen, Copenhagen, Denmark

3 Danish Cancer Society, Copenhagen, Denmark

References

[1] Lichanska AM, Waters MJ: How growth hormone controls growth, obesity and sexual dimorphism. *Trends Genet* 2008, 24(1):41–47.

[2] Moller N, Jorgensen JO: Effects of growth hormone on glucose, lipid, and protein metabolism in human subjects. *Endocr Rev* 2009, 30(2):152–177.

[3] Baik M, Yu JH, Hennighausen L: Growth hormone-STAT5 regulation of growth, hepatocellular carcinoma, and liver metabolism. *Ann NY Acad Sci* 2011, 1229:29–37.

[4] List EO, Sackmann-Sala L, Berryman DE, Funk K, Kelder B, Gosney ES, Okada S, Ding J, Cruz-Topete D, Kopchick JJ: Endocrine parameters and phenotypes of the growth hormone receptor gene disrupted (GHR-/-) mouse. *Endocr Rev* 2011, 32(3):356–386.

[5] Brooks AJ, Waters MJ: The growth hormone receptor: mechanism of activation and clinical implications. *Nat Rev Endocrinol* 2010, 6(9):515–525.

[6] Carter-Su C, Schwartz J, Argetsinger LS: Growth hormone signaling pathways. *Growth Horm IGF Res* 2016, 28:11–15.

[7] Vidal OM, Merino R, Rico-Bautista E, Fernandez-Perez L, Chia DJ, Woelfle J, Ono M, Lenhard B, Norstedt G, Rotwein P, et al.: In vivo transcript profiling and phylogenetic analysis identifies suppressor of cytokine signaling 2 as a direct signal transducer and activator of transcription 5b target in liver. *Mol Endocrinol* 2007, 21(1):293–311.

[8] Cesena TI, Cui TX, Piwien-Pilipuk G, Kaplani J, Calinescu AA, Huo JS, Iniguez-Lluhi JA, Kwok R, Schwartz J: Multiple mechanisms of growth hormone-regulated gene transcription. *Mol Genet Metab* 2007, 90(2):126–133.

[9] Wauthier V, Waxman DJ: Sex-specific early growth hormone response genes in rat liver. *Mol Endocrinol* 2008, 22(8):1962–1974.

[10] Waxman DJ, O'Connor C: Growth hormone regulation of sex-dependent liver gene expression. *Mol Endocrinol* 2006, 20(11):2613–2629.

[11] Rosenfeld RG, Kofoed E, Buckway C, Little B, Woods KA, Tsubaki J, Pratt KA, Bezrodnik L, Jasper H, Tepper A, et al.: Identification of the first patient with a confirmed mutation of the JAK-STAT system. *Pediatr Nephrol* 2005, 20(3):303–305.

[12] Walenkamp MJ, Vidarsdottir S, Pereira AM, Karperien M, van Doorn J, van Duyvenvoorde HA, Breuning MH, Roelfsema F, Kruithof MF, van Dissel J, et al.: Growth hormone secretion and immunological function of a male patient with a homozygous STAT5b mutation. *Eur J Endocrinol* 2007, 156(2):155–165.

[13] Weedon MN, Lango H, Lindgren CM, Wallace C, Evans DM, Mangino M, Freathy RM, Perry JR, Stevens S, Hall AS, et al.: Genome-wide association analysis identifies 20 loci that influence adult height. *Nat Genet* 2008, 40(5):575–583.

[14] Gudbjartsson DF, Walters GB, Thorleifsson G, Stefansson H, Halldorsson BV, Zusmanovich P, Sulem P, Thorlacius S, Gylfason A, Steinberg S, et al.: Many sequence variants affecting diversity of adult human height. *Nat Genet* 2008, 40(5):609–615.

[15] Rosenbloom AL: A half-century of studies of growth hormone insensitivity/Laron síndrome: a historical perspective. *Growth Horm IGF Res* 2016, 28:46–50.

[16] Flores-Morales A, Greenhalgh CJ, Norstedt G, Rico-Bautista E: Negative regulation of growth hormone receptor signaling. *Mol Endocrinol* 2006, 20(2):241–253.

[17] Mode A, Gustafsson JA: Sex and the liver—a journey through five decades. *Drug Metab Rev* 2006, 38(1–2):197–207.

[18] da Silva Almeida AC, Strous GJ, van Rossum AG: BetaTrCP controls GH receptor degradation via two different motifs. *Mol Endocrinol* 2012, 26(1):165–177.

[19] Rico-Bautista E, Flores-Morales A, Fernandez-Perez L: Suppressor of cytokine signaling (SOCS) 2, a protein with multiple functions. *Cytokine Growth Factor Rev* 2006, 17(6): 431–439.

[20] Linossi EM, Babon JJ, Hilton DJ, Nicholson SE: Suppression of cytokine signaling: the SOCS perspective. *Cytokine Growth Factor Rev* 2013, 24(3):241–248.

[21] Greenhalgh CJ, Rico-Bautista E, Lorentzon M, Thaus AL, Morgan PO, Willson TA, Zervoudakis P, Metcalf D, Street I, Nicola NA, et al.: SOCS2 negatively regulates growth hormone action in vitro and in vivo. *J Clin Invest* 2005, 115(2):397–406.

[22] Uyttendaele I, Lemmens I, Verhee A, De Smet AS, Vandekerckhove J, Lavens D, Peelman F, Tavernier J: Mammalian protein-protein interaction trap (MAPPIT) analysis of STAT5, CIS, and SOCS2 interactions with the growth hormone receptor. *Mol Endocrinol* 2007, 21(11):2821–2831.

[23] Zhou W, Wei W, Sun Y: Genetically engineered mouse models for functional studies of SKP1-CUL1-F-box-protein (SCF) E3 ubiquitin ligases. *Cell Res* 2013, 23(5):599–619.

[24] Vesterlund M, Zadjali F, Persson T, Nielsen ML, Kessler BM, Norstedt G, Flores-Morales A: The SOCS2 ubiquitin ligase complex regulates growth hormone receptor levels. *PLoS One* 2011, 6(9):e25358.

[25] da Silva Almeida AC, Hocking HG, Boelens R, Strous GJ, van Rossum AG: BetaTrCP interacts with the ubiquitin-dependent endocytosis motif of the GH receptor in an unconventional manner. *Biochem J* 2013, 453(2):291–301.

[26] Zadjali F, Santana-Farre R, Vesterlund M, Carow B, Mirecki-Garrido M, Hernandez-Hernandez I, Flodstrom-Tullberg M, Parini P, Rottenberg M, Norstedt G, et al.: SOCS2 deletion protects against hepatic steatosis but worsens insulin resistance in high-fat-diet-fed mice. *FASEB J* 2012, 26(8):3282–3291.

[27] Tollet-Egnell P, Flores-Morales A, Stavreus-Evers A, Sahlin L, Norstedt G: Growth hormone regulation of SOCS-2, SOCS-3, and CIS messenger ribonucleic acid expression in the rat. *Endocrinology* 1999, 140(8):3693–3704.

[28] Greenhalgh CJ, Alexander WS: Suppressors of cytokine signalling and regulation of growth hormone action. *Growth Horm IGF Res* 2004, 14(3):200–206.

[29] Michaylira CZ, Simmons JG, Ramocki NM, Scull BP, McNaughton KK, Fuller CR, Lund PK: Suppressor of cytokine signaling-2 limits intestinal growth and enterotrophic actions of IGF-I in vivo. *Am J Physiol Gastrointest Liver Physiol* 2006, 291(3):G472–G481.

[30] Adams TE, Hansen JA, Starr R, Nicola NA, Hilton DJ, Billestrup N: Growth hormone preferentially induces the rapid, transient expression of SOCS-3, a novel inhibitor of cytokine receptor signaling. *J Biol Chem* 1998, 273(3):1285–1287.

[31] Hansen JA, Lindberg K, Hilton DJ, Nielsen JH, Billestrup N: Mechanism of inhibition of growth hormone receptor signaling by suppressor of cytokine signaling proteins. *Mol Endocrinol* 1999, 13(11):1832–1843.

[32] Yasukawa H, Sasaki A, Yoshimura A: Negative regulation of cytokine signaling pathways. *Annu Rev Immunol* 2000, 18:143–164.

[33] Alexander WS, Starr R, Metcalf D, Nicholson SE, Farley A, Elefanty AG, Brysha M, Kile BT, Richardson R, Baca M, et al.: Suppressors of cytokine signaling (SOCS): negative regulators of signal transduction. *J Leukoc Biol* 1999, 66(4):588–592.

[34] Turnley AM: Role of SOCS2 in growth hormone actions. *Trends Endocrinol Metab* 2005, 16(2):53–58.

[35] Leung KC, Waters MJ, Markus I, Baumbach WR, Ho KK: Insulin and insulin-like growth factor-I acutely inhibit surface translocation of growth hormone receptors in osteoblasts: a novel mechanism of growth hormone receptor regulation. *Proc Natl Acad Sci USA* 1997, 94(21):11381–11386.

[36] De Rocca Serra-Nedelec A, Edouard T, Treguer K, Tajan M, Araki T, Dance M, Mus M, Montagner A, Tauber M, Salles JP, et al.: Noonan syndrome-causing SHP2 mutants inhibit insulin-like growth factor 1 release via growth hormone-induced ERK hyper-activation, which contributes to short stature. *Proc Natl Acad Sci USA* 2012, 109(11):4257–4262.

[37] Ehlting C, Bohmer O, Hahnel MJ, Thomas M, Zanger UM, Gaestel M, Knoefel WT, Schulte Am Esch J, Haussinger D, Bode JG: Oncostatin M regulates SOCS3 mRNA stability via the MEK-ERK1/2-pathway independent of p38(MAPK)/MK2. *Cell Signal* 2015, 27(3):555–567.

[38] Ram PA, Waxman DJ: Interaction of growth hormone-activated STATs with SH2-containing phosphotyrosine phosphatase SHP-1 and nuclear JAK2 tyrosine kinase. *J Biol Chem* 1997, 272(28):17694–17702.

[39] Hackett RH, Wang YD, Sweitzer S, Feldman G, Wood WI, Larner AC: Mapping of a cytoplasmic domain of the human growth hormone receptor that regulates rates of inactivation of Jak2 and Stat proteins. *J Biol Chem* 1997, 272(17):11128–11132.

[40] Gu F, Dube N, Kim JW, Cheng A, Ibarra-Sanchez Mde J, Tremblay ML, Boisclair YR: Protein tyrosine phosphatase 1B attenuates growth hormone-mediated JAK2-STAT signaling. *Mol Cell Biol* 2003, 23(11):3753–3762.

[41] Pasquali C, Curchod ML, Walchli S, Espanel X, Guerrier M, Arigoni F, Strous G, Hooft van Huijsduijnen R: Identification of protein tyrosine phosphatases with specificity for the ligand-activated growth hormone receptor *Mol Endocrinol* 2003, 17(11):2228–2239.

[42] Le Roith D, Bondy C, Yakar S, Liu JL, Butler A: The somatomedin hypothesis: 2001. *Endocr Rev* 2001, 22(1):53–74.

[43] Kaplan SA, Cohen P: The somatomedin hypothesis 2007: 50 years later. *J Clin Endocrinol Metab* 2007, 92(12):4529–4535.

[44] Lupu F, Terwilliger JD, Lee K, Segre GV, Efstratiadis A: Roles of growth hormone and insulin-like growth factor 1 in mouse postnatal growth. *Dev Biol* 2001, 229(1):141–162.

[45] Giustina A, Mazziotti G, Canalis E: Growth hormone, insulin-like growth factors, and the skeleton. *Endocr Rev* 2008, 29(5):535–559.

[46] Hutchison MR, Bassett MH, White PC: Insulin-like growth factor-I and fibroblast growth factor, but not growth hormone, affect growth plate chondrocyte proliferation. *Endocrinology* 2007, 148(7):3122–3130.

[47] Yakar S, Liu JL, Stannard B, Butler A, Accili D, Sauer B, LeRoith D: Normal growth and development in the absence of hepatic insulin-like growth factor I. *Proc Natl Acad Sci USA* 1999, 96(13):7324–7329.

[48] Liu JL, Yakar S, LeRoith D: Conditional knockout of mouse insulin-like growth factor-1 gene using the Cre/loxP system. *Proc Soc Exp Biol Med* 2000, 223(4):344–351.

[49] Stratikopoulos E, Szabolcs M, Dragatsis I, Klinakis A, Efstratiadis A: The hormonal action of IGF1 in postnatal mouse growth. *Proc Natl Acad Sci USA* 2008, 105(49):19378–19383.

[50] Le Roith D, Scavo L, Butler A: What is the role of circulating IGF-I? *Trends Endocrinol Metab* 2001, 12(2):48–52.

[51] Udy GB, Towers RP, Snell RG, Wilkins RJ, Park SH, Ram PA, Waxman DJ, Davey HW: Requirement of STAT5b for sexual dimorphism of body growth rates and liver gene expression. *Proc Natl Acad Sci USA* 1997, 94(14):7239–7244.

[52] Mueller KM, Themanns M, Friedbichler K, Kornfeld JW, Esterbauer H, Tuckermann JP, Moriggl R: Hepatic growth hormone and glucocorticoid receptor signaling in body growth, steatosis and metabolic liver cancer development. *Mol Cell Endocrinol* 2012, 361(1–2):1–11.

[53] Bjornstrom L, Sjoberg M: Mechanisms of estrogen receptor signaling: convergence of genomic and nongenomic actions on target genes. *Mol Endocrinol* 2005, 19(4):833–842.

[54] Klover P, Hennighausen L: Postnatal body growth is dependent on the transcription factors signal transducers and activators of transcription 5a/b in muscle: a role for autocrine/paracrine insulin-like growth factor I. *Endocrinology* 2007, 148(4):1489–1497.

[55] Leroith D, Nissley P: Knock your SOCS off! *J Clin Invest* 2005, 115(2):233–236.

[56] Greenhalgh CJ, Bertolino P, Asa SL, Metcalf D, Corbin JE, Adams TE, Davey HW, Nicola NA, Hilton DJ, Alexander WS: Growth enhancement in suppressor of cytokine signaling 2 (SOCS-2)-deficient mice is dependent on signal transducer and activator of transcription 5b (STAT5b). *Mol Endocrinol* 2002, 16(6):1394–1406.

[57] Horvat S, Medrano JF: Lack of Socs2 expression causes the high-growth phenotype in mice. *Genomics* 2001, 72(2):209–212.

[58] Greenhalgh CJ, Metcalf D, Thaus AL, Corbin JE, Uren R, Morgan PO, Fabri LJ, Zhang JG, Martin HM, Willson TA, et al.: Biological evidence that SOCS-2 can act either as an enhancer or suppressor of growth hormone signaling. *J Biol Chem* 2002, 277(43):40181–40184.

[59] Kiu H, Greenhalgh CJ, Thaus A, Hilton DJ, Nicola NA, Alexander WS, Roberts AW: Regulation of multiple cytokine signalling pathways by SOCS3 is independent of SOCS2. *Growth Factors* 2009, 27(6):384–393.

[60] Parks JS, Brown MR, Faase ME: The spectrum of growth-hormone insensitivity. *J Pediatr* 1997, 131(1 Pt 2):S45–S50.

[61] Wassenaar MJ, Dekkers OM, Pereira AM, Wit JM, Smit JW, Biermasz NR, Romijn JA: Impact of the exon 3-deleted growth hormone (GH) receptor polymorphism on baseline height and the growth response to recombinant human GH therapy in GH-deficient (GHD) and non-GHD children with short stature: a systematic review and meta-analysis. *J Clin Endocrinol Metab* 2009, 94(10):3721–3730.

[62] Renehan AG, Solomon M, Zwahlen M, Morjaria R, Whatmore A, Audi L, Binder G, Blum W, Bougneres P, Santos CD, et al.: Growth hormone receptor polymorphism and growth hormone therapy response in children: a Bayesian meta-analysis. *Am J Epidemiol* 2012, 175(9):867–877.

[63] Braz AF, Costalonga EF, Montenegro LR, Trarbach EB, Antonini SR, Malaquias AC, Ramos ES, Mendonca BB, Arnhold IJ, Jorge AA: The interactive effect of GHR-exon 3 and -202 A/C IGFBP3 polymorphisms on rhGH responsiveness and treatment outcomes in patients with Turner syndrome. *J Clin Endocrinol Metab* 2012, 97(4):E671–E677.

[64] Costalonga EF, Antonini SR, Guerra G, Jr., Coletta RR, Franca MM, Braz AF, Mendonca BB, Arnhold IJ, Jorge AA: Growth hormone pharmacogenetics: the interactive effect of a microsatellite in the IGF1 promoter region with the GHR-exon 3 and -202 A/C IGFBP3 variants on treatment outcomes of children with severe GH deficiency. *Pharmacogenomics J* 2012, 12(5):439–445.

[65] Chan Y, Holmen OL, Dauber A, Vatten L, Havulinna AS, Skorpen F, Kvaloy K, Silander K, Nguyen TT, Willer C, et al.: Common variants show predicted polygenic effects on height in the tails of the distribution, except in extremely short individuals. *PLoS Genet* 2011, 7(12):e1002439.

[66] Braz AF, Costalonga EF, Trarbach EB, Scalco RC, Malaquias AC, Guerra-Junior G, Antonini SR, Mendonca BB, Arnhold IJ, Jorge AA: Genetic predictors of long-term response to growth hormone (GH) therapy in children with GH deficiency and Turner syndrome: the influence of a SOCS2 polymorphism. *J Clin Endocrinol Metab* 2014, 99(9):E1808–E1813.

[67] Sovio U, Bennett AJ, Millwood IY, Molitor J, O'Reilly PF, Timpson NJ, Kaakinen M, Laitinen J, Haukka J, Pillas D, et al.: Genetic determinants of height growth assessed longitudinally from infancy to adulthood in the northern Finland birth cohort 1966. *PLoS Genet* 2009, 5(3):e1000409.

[68] Metcalf D, Greenhalgh CJ, Viney E, Willson TA, Starr R, Nicola NA, Hilton DJ, Alexander WS: Gigantism in mice lacking suppressor of cytokine signalling-2. *Nature* 2000, 405(6790):1069–1073.

[69] Ohlsson C, Bengtsson BA, Isaksson OG, Andreassen TT, Slootweg MC: Growth hormone and bone. *Endocr Rev* 1998, 19(1):55–79.

[70] Andreassen TT, Oxlund H: The effects of growth hormone on cortical and cancellous bone. *J Musculoskelet Neuronal Interact* 2001, 2(1):49–58.

[71] Metcalf D, Alexander WS, Elefanty AG, Nicola NA, Hilton DJ, Starr R, Mifsud S, Di Rago L: Aberrant hematopoiesis in mice with inactivation of the gene encoding SOCS-1. *Leukemia* 1999, 13(6):926–934.

[72] Macrae VE, Horvat S, Pells SC, Dale H, Collinson RS, Pitsillides AA, Ahmed SF, Farquharson C: Increased bone mass, altered trabecular architecture and modified growth plate organization in the growing skeleton of SOCS2 deficient mice. *J Cell Physiol* 2009, 218(2):276–284.

[73] Lorentzon M, Greenhalgh CJ, Mohan S, Alexander WS, Ohlsson C: Reduced bone mineral density in SOCS-2-deficient mice. *Pediatr Res* 2005, 57(2):223–226.

[74] Dobie R, Ahmed SF, Staines KA, Pass C, Jasim S, MacRae VE, Farquharson C: Increased linear bone growth by GH in the absence of SOCS2 is independent of IGF-1. *J Cell Physiol* 2015, 230(11):2796–2806.

[75] Vestergaard PF, Vendelbo MH, Pedersen SB, Juul A, Ringgard S, Moller N, Jessen N, Jorgensen JO: GH signaling in skeletal muscle and adipose tissue in healthy human subjects: impact of gender and age. *Eur J Endocrinol* 2014, 171(5):623–631.

[76] Clasen BF, Poulsen MM, Escande C, Pedersen SB, Moller N, Chini EN, Jessen N, Jorgensen JO: Growth hormone signaling in muscle and adipose tissue of obese human subjects: associations with measures of body composition and interaction with resveratrol treatment. *J Clin Endocrinol Metab* 2014, 99(12):E2565–E2573.

[77] Resmini E, Morte B, Sorianello E, Gallardo E, de Luna N, Illa I, Zorzano A, Bernal J, Webb SM: Identification of novel GH-regulated genes in C2C12 cells. *Horm Metab Res* 2011, 43(13):919–930.

[78] Ouyang X, Fujimoto M, Nakagawa R, Serada S, Tanaka T, Nomura S, Kawase I, Kishimoto T, Naka T: SOCS-2 interferes with myotube formation and potentiates osteoblast differentiation through upregulation of JunB in C2C12 cells. *J Cell Physiol* 2006, 207(2):428–436.

[79] Gan L, Liu Z, Zhang Z, Yang X, Liu J, Sun C: SOCS2 inhibited mitochondria biogenesis via inhibiting p38 MAPK/ATF2 pathway in C2C12 cells. *Mol Biol Rep* 2014, 41(2):627–637.

[80] Barclay JL, Nelson CN, Ishikawa M, Murray LA, Kerr LM, McPhee TR, Powell EE, Waters MJ: GH-dependent STAT5 signaling plays an important role in hepatic lipid metabolism. *Endocrinology* 2011, 152(1):181–192.

[81] Sos BC, Harris C, Nordstrom SM, Tran JL, Balazs M, Caplazi P, Febbraio M, Applegate MA, Wagner KU, Weiss EJ: Abrogation of growth hormone secretion rescues fatty liver in mice with hepatocyte-specific deletion of JAK2. *J Clin Invest* 2011, 121(4):1412–1423.

[82] Fan Y, Fang X, Tajima A, Geng X, Ranganathan S, Dong H, Trucco M, Sperling MA: Evolution of hepatic steatosis to fibrosis and adenoma formation in liver-specific growth hormone receptor knockout mice. *Front Endocrinol (Lausanne)* 2014, 5:218.

[83] Klover P, Chen W, Zhu BM, Hennighausen L: Skeletal muscle growth and fiber composition in mice are regulated through the transcription factors STAT5a/b: linking growth hormone to the androgen receptor. *FASEB J* 2009, 23(9):3140–3148.

[84] Iglesias-Gato D, Chuan YC, Wikstrom P, Augsten S, Jiang N, Niu Y, Seipel A, Danneman D, Vermeij M, Fernandez-Perez L, et al.: SOCS2 mediates the cross talk between androgen and growth hormone signaling in prostate cancer. *Carcinogenesis* 2014, 35(1): 24–33.

[85] Vidarsdottir S, Walenkamp MJ, Pereira AM, Karperien M, van Doorn J, van Duyvenvoorde HA, White S, Breuning MH, Roelfsema F, Kruithof MF, et al.: Clinical and biochemical characteristics of a male patient with a novel homozygous STAT5b mutation. *J Clin Endocrinol Metab* 2006, 91(9):3482–3485.

[86] Hong C, Tontonoz P: Liver X receptors in lipid metabolism: opportunities for drug discovery. *Nat Rev Drug Discov* 2014, 13(6):433–444.

[87] Zadjali F, Santana-Farre R, Mirecki-Garrido M, Ellis E, Norstedt G, Fernandez-Perez L, Flores-Morales A: Liver X receptor agonist downregulates growth hormone signaling in the liver. *Horm Mol Biol Clin Investig* 2011, 8(2):471–478.

[88] Al Kharusi A, Mirecki-Garrido M, Ma Z, Zadjali F, Flores-Morales A, Nystrom T, Castrillo A, Bjorklund A, Norstedt G, Fernandez-Perez L. Suppressor of cytokine signaling 2 (SOCS2) deletion protects against multiple low dose-streptozotocin-induced type I diabetes in adult male mice. *Horm Mol Biol Clin Investig* 2016, 26(1):67–76.

[89] Galic S, Sachithanandan N, Kay TW, Steinberg GR: Suppressor of cytokine signalling (SOCS) proteins as guardians of inflammatory responses critical for regulating insulin sensitivity. *Biochem J* 2014, 461(2):177–188.

[90] Rupp R, Senin P, Sarry J, Allain C, Tasca C, Ligat L, Portes D, Woloszyn F, Bouchez O, Tabouret G, et al.: Apoint mutation in suppressor of cytokine signalling 2 (Socs2) increases the susceptibility to inflammation of the mammary gland while associated with higher body weight and size and higher milk production in a sheep model. *PLoS Genet* 2015, 11(12):e1005629.

[91] Vitali C, Bassani C, Chiodoni C, Fellini E, Guarnotta C, Miotti S, Sangaletti S, Fuligni F, De Cecco L, Piccaluga PP, et al.: SOCS2 controls proliferation and stemness of hematopoietic cells under stress conditions and its deregulation marks unfavorable acute leukemias. *Cancer Res* 2015, 75(11):2387–2399.

[92] Newton VA, Ramocki NM, Scull BP, Simmons JG, McNaughton K, Lund PK: Suppressor of cytokine signaling-2 gene disruption promotes Apc(Min/+) tumorigenesis and activator protein-1 activation. *Am J Pathol* 2010, 176(5):2320–2332.

[93] Michaylira CZ, Ramocki NM, Simmons JG, Tanner CK, McNaughton KK, Woosley JT, Greenhalgh CJ, Lund PK: Haplotype insufficiency for suppressor of cytokine signaling-2 enhances intestinal growth and promotes polyp formation in growth hormone-transgenic mice. *Endocrinology* 2006, 147(4):1632–1641.

[94] Kerrigan JR, Rogol AD: The impact of gonadal steroid hormone action on growth hormone secretion during childhood and adolescence. *Endocr Rev* 1992, 13(2):281–298.

[95] Mauvais-Jarvis F: Estrogen and androgen receptors: regulators of fuel homeostasis and emerging targets for diabetes and obesity. *Trends Endocrinol Metab* 2011, 22(1):24–33.

[96] Fisher B, Gunduz N, Saffer EA, Zheng S: Relation of estrogen and its receptor to rat liver growth and regeneration. *Cancer Res* 1984, 44(6):2410–2415.

[97] Vidal O, Lindberg MK, Hollberg K, Baylink DJ, Andersson G, Lubahn DB, Mohan S, Gustafsson JA, Ohlsson C: Estrogen receptor specificity in the regulation of skeletal growth and maturation in male mice. *Proc Natl Acad Sci USA* 2000, 97(10):5474–5479.

[98] Meinhardt UJ, Ho KK: Modulation of growth hormone action by sex steroids. *Clin Endocrinol (Oxf)* 2006, 65(4):413–422.

[99] Weissberger AJ, Ho KK: Activation of the somatotropic axis by testosterone in adult males: evidence for the role of aromatization. *J Clin Endocrinol Metab* 1993, 76(6): 1407–1412.

[100] Giustina A, Scalvini T, Tassi C, Desenzani P, Poiesi C, Wehrenberg WB, Rogol AD, Veldhuis JD: Maturation of the regulation of growth hormone secretion in young males with hypogonadotropic hypogonadism pharmacologically exposed to progressive increments in serum testosterone. *J Clin Endocrinol Metab* 1997, 82(4):1210–1219.

[101] Jospe N, Orlowski CC, Furlanetto RW: Comparison of transdermal and oral estrogen therapy in girls with Turner's syndrome. *J Pediatr Endocrinol Metab* 1995, 8(2):111–116.

[102] Mansfield MJ, Rudlin CR, Crigler JF, Jr., Karol KA, Crawford JD, Boepple PA, Crowley WF, Jr.: Changes in growth and serum growth hormone and plasma somatomedin-C levels during suppression of gonadal sex steroid secretion in girls with central precocious puberty. *J Clin Endocrinol Metab* 1988, 66(1):3–9.

[103] Perry RJ, Farquharson C, Ahmed SF: The role of sex steroids in controlling pubertal growth. *Clin Endocrinol (Oxf)* 2008, 68(1):4–15.

[104] Venken K, Schuit F, Van Lommel L, Tsukamoto K, Kopchick JJ, Coschigano K, Ohlsson C, Moverare S, Boonen S, Bouillon R, et al.: Growth without growth hormone receptor: estradiol is a major growth hormone-independent regulator of hepatic IGF-I synthesis. *J Bone Miner Res* 2005, 20(12):2138–2149.

[105] Drop SL, De Waal WJ, De Muinck Keizer-Schrama SM: Sex steroid treatment of constitutionally tall stature. *Endocr Rev* 1998, 19(5):540–558.

[106] Weise M, De-Levi S, Barnes KM, Gafni RI, Abad V, Baron J: Effects of estrogen on growth plate senescence and epiphyseal fusion. *Proc Natl Acad Sci USA* 2001, 98(12):6871–6876.

[107] Ross JL, Cassorla FG, Skerda MC, Valk IM, Loriaux DL, Cutler GB, Jr.: A preliminary study of the effect of estrogen dose on growth in Turner's syndrome. *N Engl J Med* 1983, 309(18):1104–1106.

[108] Goldzieher MA: Treatment of excessive growth in the adolescent female. *J Clin Endocrinol Metab* 1956, 16(2):249–252.

[109] Frank GR: The role of estrogen in pubertal skeletal physiology: epiphyseal maturation and mineralization of the skeleton. *Acta Paediatr* 1995, 84(6):627–630.

[110] Leung KC, Doyle N, Ballesteros M, Sjogren K, Watts CK, Low TH, Leong GM, Ross RJ, Ho KK: Estrogen inhibits GH signaling by suppressing GH-induced JAK2 phosphorylation, an effect mediated by SOCS-2. *Proc Natl Acad Sci USA* 2003, 100(3):1016–1021.

[111] Bolamperti S, Mrak E, Moro G, Sirtori P, Fraschini G, Guidobono F, Rubinacci A, Villa I: 17beta-Estradiol positively modulates growth hormone signaling through the reduction of SOCS2 negative feedback in human osteoblasts. *Bone* 2013, 55(1):84–92.

Chapter 6

Mannose-6-Phosphate/Insulin-Like Growth Factor 2 Receptor (M6P/IGF2-R) in Growth and Disease: A Review

Guy Joseph Lemamy, Bénédicte Ndeboko,
Serge Thierry Omouessi and Justine Mouecoucou

Additional information is available at the end of the chapter

http://dx.doi.org/10.5772/64810

Abstract

This work aims to summarize the current knowledge about Mannose-6- Phosphate/ Insulin-like Growth Factor 2 Receptor (M6P/IGF2-R) in the regulation of growth and development, and its involvement in tumor progression. M6P/IGF2-R binds both molecules sharing M6P signals and IGF2. The studies showed that M6P/IGF2-R is involved in the trafficking of mannnose-6-phosphorylated enzymes from the Trans-Golgi Network (TGN) to lysosomes and the uptake of secreted proenzymes from the plasma membrane to the lysosomes via clathrin-coated vesicles for their maturation. The M6P/IGF2-R acts as a scavenger that binds IGF2 and transports it to lysosomes for its degradation since IGF2 exerts its biological effects on cell proliferation and development by binding with lower affinity on IGF1 receptor, which is structurally similar to insulin receptor and different from the M6P/IGF2-R. The M6P/IGF2-R has also been studied in human cancer, and frequent losses of heterozygosity (LOH) at the 6q25-27 gene region with mutations in the remaining allele have been described. These results led to consider M6P/IGF2-R gene as a putative tumor suppressor and its potential prognostic value has been suggested.

Keywords: M6P/IGF2-R, genomic imprinting, cell growth and development, loss of heterozygosity (LOH), human cancer, tumor suppressor

1. Introduction

Two mannose-6-phosphate receptors (M6PRs) have been described: the mannose-6-phosphate/insulin-like growth factor 2 receptor (M6P/IGF2-R) binds both M6P ligands and IGF2 [1, 2] and the cation-dependent mannose-6-phosphate receptor (CD-M6PR), which needs divalent cations to bind M6P ligands but does not bind insulin-like growth factor 2 [3]. The M6P/IGF2-R is also called cation-independent M6P receptor (CI-M6PR) because it does not need ions to bind its ligands. In comparison to their molecular weight, the CD-M6PR (46 kDa) and the CI-M6PR (250 kDa) are, respectively, called "Small" and "Big" M6P receptor.

Historically, the insulin-like growth factors have been predicted by studying the action of the pituitary growth hormone (GH) on the growth. GH is a pleiotropic hormone secreted by the pituitary gland, which acts as a growth factor on bone and muscle tissues, or as a differentiation factor and a metabolic regulator in liver, fat, and muscle tissues. GH has been historically proposed to act by using intermediates, the somatomedins, which were able to exert growth hormone-like effects on the skeletal cartilage and other tissues [4]. Further analyses revealed two molecules sharing high homology with proinsulin that were consequently called IGF1 and IGF2 [5, 6].

The insulin-like growth factors 1 and 2 have similar biological effects, but there are nevertheless differences in their expression. In mammals, IGF1 is preferentially expressed after birth and is almost exclusively produced in the liver, whereas IGF2 is preferentially expressed in early stages of embryonic and fetal development in many tissues. In adults, IGF2 is expressed not only in liver but also in other tissues such as the brain (essentially the meninges) and choroid plexus [7]. IGFs play an important role in the regulation of normal cell growth and proliferation, or in malignant transformation [8, 9].

The growth hormone's receptor is a single transmembrane protein sharing similarities with the prolactin receptor and, to a lesser extent, with some members of cytokine receptor family. The binding of GH to its receptor induces signaling pathways in most target cells to transduce hormonal message to the nucleus, which results to activate the transcription of a variety of genes coding for IGFs or several other proteins such as transcription factors, hormones, hormone receptors, prolactin receptor, c-fos, cytochrome P450 IIC, and various enzymes. Several studies reported that M6P/IGF2-R is involved in tumor development in human [9].

This chapter discusses the role of the M6P/IGF2-R in the regulation of growth and its involvement in tumor progression.

2. Structure of the M6P/IGF2-R

The mannose-6-phosphate/insulin-like growth factor 2 is a single-chain transmembrane protein, of 250–300 kDa that functions as a multifunctional receptor by binding molecules sharing M6P signals and IGF2 [1, 2]. The M6P/IGF2-R contains 2451 amino acids with a large extracellular domain made of 2264 residues, a short transmembrane domain of 23 residues, and a small cytoplasmic domain of 164 residues. The extracellular domain of M6P/IGF2-R consists of a 40-residue amino acid signal sequence and 15 conserved repeat domains. Each repeat contains an average length of 150 residues and 13–37% amino acids identity rich in cysteine residues, which make it highly conserved throughout species, with 60–90% homology (**Table 1**). The repeat number 13 contains a 43-amino acid sequence homologous to the

http://dx.doi.org/10.5772/64810

collagen-binding domain type 2-region of fibronectin. The mannose-6-phoshate signals bind to repeats 3 and 9, whereas IGF2 binds to repeat 11 [10–12]. The M6P signals bind to residues R^{435} and R^{1334} localized, respectively, in domains 3 and 9 [10], and the residues (Q^{392}-S^{431}-E^{460}-Y^{465}) localized in repeat 3 and (Q^{1292}-H^{1329}-E^{1354}-Y^{1360}) localized in repeat 9 play an essential role in M6P recognition [13] (**Figure 1**). Further studies showed that domain 5 also steps in mannose-6-phosphate signal binding. The amino acid residues 1508–1566 localized in repeat 11 are needed for IGF2 binding [14]. Moreover, the affinity of IGF2 binding is enhanced by the fibronectin type 2-like insert of domain 13, though the biochemical mechanisms of that enhancement are unknown [9]. However, mannose-6-phosphate receptor does not bind to IGF2 in oviparous [15].

	Human	Bovine	Chicken	Mouse
Human	100	90	60	89
Bovine	90	100	60	87
Chicken	60	60	100	–
Mouse	89	87	–	100

The M6P/IGF2-R amino acid sequences have been compared. Results, expressed in percentage, showed high homology throughout species including human and varies from 60 to 90%.

Table 1. Sequence homology of M6P/IGF2-R in animals.

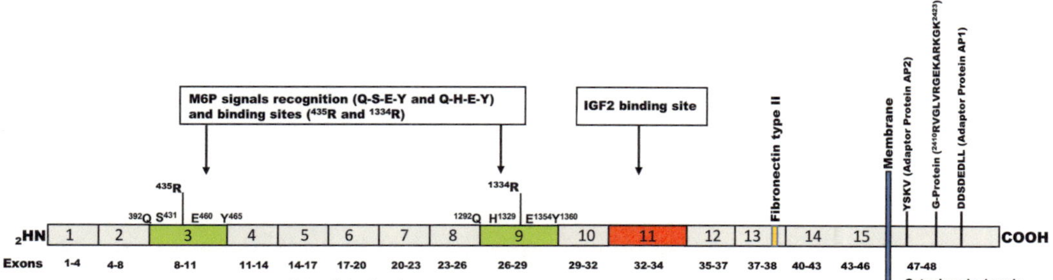

Figure 1. Structure and gene organization of mouse M6P/IGF2 receptor. Numbers in boxes (1–15) symbolize the repeat domains. Binding sites are indicated in repeats 3 and 9 (for M6P signals) and in repeat 11 (for IGF2). M6P/IGF2-R gene consists of 48 exons encoding for the full-length receptor. Amino acid sequences of cytoplasmic domain have been suggested to interact with adaptor or G proteins.

The M6P/IGF2-R has been shown to be shed from the cell surface and secreted in the culture medium in Michigan Cancer Foundation 7 (MCF7) cancer cell lines [16] Moreover, other studies described the M6P/IGF2-R as a circulating protein in rat [17] or in human serum and urine [18]. Subsequent studies showed that the serum form of M6P/IGF2-R is truncated or altered in its cytoplasmic domain with a molecular weight of less than 250 kDa [19].

2.1. Genomic organization and gene imprinting

In mice, M6P/IGF2-R is coded by chromosome 17 [20]. The gene contains 48 exons (**Figure 1**) and spreads on 93 kb [21]. M6P/IGF2-R is imprinted in mice. Genomic imprinting is a developmental gene regulation whereby only one of the parental alleles is expressed [9].

In mice, the M6P/IGF2-R is exclusively expressed from the allele inherited from the mother, while IGF2 is expressed from the allele inherited from the father [9]. The imprinting of M6P/IGF2-R is regulated by the intron 2-region in paternal allele, which contains an antisense transcript mediating the silencing of the paternal M6P/IGF2-R allele. Deletion of that intron 2-region disrupts the silencing and leads to biallelic expression of M6P/IGF2-R inherited from the father [22]. Mice inherited from a disrupted M6P/IGF2-R gene from their mother do not express the receptor in tissues and show malformations in lungs and cardiac muscle. By contrast, when the same gene is inherited from the father, no abnormality was observed in the development confirming the paternal imprinting of the M6P/IGF2-R gene [23].

The oppositely imprinting of IGF2 and M6P/IGF2-R genes supposes that M6P/IGF2-R produced from the mother acts as a scavenger, which neutralizes IGF2 produced from the father before it reaches the signaling from IGF1 or insulin receptors to exert its biological effects [9].

In human, the M6P/IGF2-R gene was previously described to map on chromosome 6q25–27 [20]. Kalscheuer et al. [24] reported that M6P/IGF2-R is not imprinted in human. Others hypothesized that such an imprinting has been probably lost during evolution [25]. Studies reporting M6P/IGF2-R imprinting as being polymorphic in human are controversial as the 3'-untranslated region (3'UTR) polymorphisms used are difficult to amplify and are subject to misinterpretation.

The consensus retained is that the receptor expression is biallelic in most humans and only less than 10% of individuals exhibit imprinting of M6P/IGF2-R [26].

3. Functions of the M6P/IGF2-R

The M6P/IGF2-R mainly and continuously circulates and cycles between endomembrane compartments and cell surface. At a steady state, it is majorly localized in trans-Golgi network (TGN) and endosomal compartments and poorly present on the plasma membrane.

3.1. Mannose-6-phosphorylated ligand binding and lysosomal enzyme routing

The mannose-6-phosphate signals bind to domains 3 and 9 [10, 12], whereas IGF2 binds to domain 11 [10, 14]. The binding affinity of M6P/IGF2-R for M6P ligands varies from Kd = 10^{-10} to 10^{-6} M and depends on phosphorylated ligand structures [27, 28]. The arginine residues ^{435}R and ^{1334}R, respectively, localized on repeats 3 and 9 are needed for M6P signal binding.

The M6P/IGF2-R is involved in the intracellular trafficking of newly synthesized mannose-6-phosphorylated lysosomal enzymes from the trans-Golgi network to the late endosomes [29,

30] and cellular uptake of secreted lysosomal enzyme precursors [31]. Lysosomal enzymes are recognized by their M6P signals and bind to M6P/IGF2-R. Adaptor proteins AP1 interact with guanosine triphosphate (GTP)ase adenosine diphosphate (ADP) ribosylation factor (ARF) and a specific sequence DDSDEDLL localized in the cytoplasmic domain of the M6P/IGF2-R [32, 33]. GTP hydrolysis-released energy is used for clathrin molecule recruitment. Lysosomal enzymes are then transported, *via* clathrin-coated vesicles, to acidified endosomal compartments where the low pH (3–5) leads to the dissociation of the enzyme from the receptor [29]. Enzymes are then released to their lysosomal final destination, the lysosomes, whereas the M6P/IGF2-R are recycled to the cell membrane or headed back to the trans-Golgi network to accomplish other transport cycles (**Figure 2**) [29].

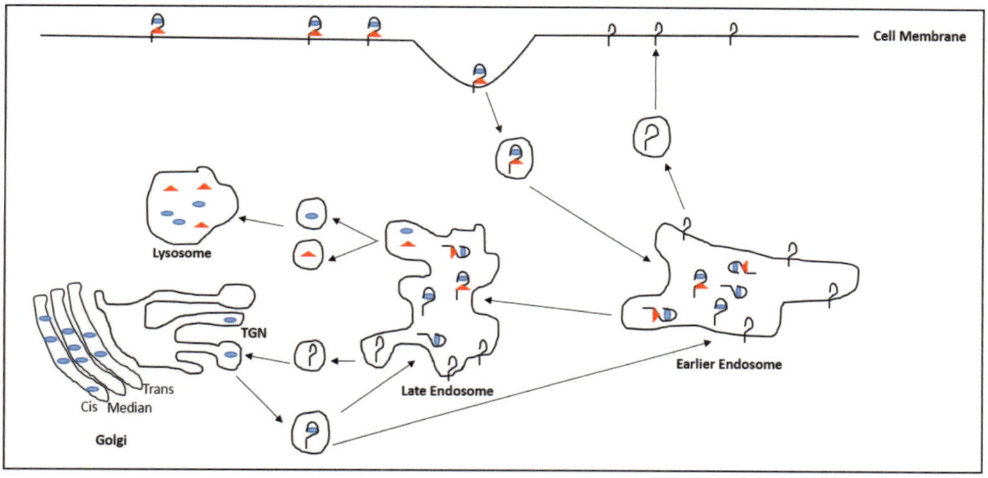

Figure 2. Endocytosis and lysosomal enzymes trafficking by the M6P/IGF2-R. Lysosomal enzymes are synthesized in endoplasmic reticulum and transported in the Golgi where they acquire M6P signals (⬬). Mannose-6-phosphorylated enzymes bind to the M6P/IGF2-R in the trans-Golgi network and are routed to the late or earlier endosomes. The receptors bound to secreted enzymes and to IGF2 (▲) at the cell membrane level are endocytosed and directed to endosomes. Enzymes and IGF2 are directed to the lysosomes and the receptors are recycled to the cell membrane.

3.2. Endocytosis of receptors and secreted proenzymes

About 10% of M6P/IGF2-R are found at the plasma membrane level and they can be internalized and recycled independently of the binding of ligand [34], whereas most of membrane receptors are internalized after the binding of their specific ligand. Secreted proenzymes are uptaken by the membrane M6P/IGF2-R and the proenzymes/M6P/IGF2-R complexes are internalized in clathrin-coated vesicles *via* an interaction between the receptor and adaptor proteins AP2 [33], which recognize cytosolic signals ^{26}YSKV^{29} of M6P/IGF2-R [35, 36]. Enzyme/receptor complexes are transported to early endosomes, the enzymes are then released and transported to late endosomes, then to lysosomes for their maturation into active enzymes, whereas the M6P/IGF2-R are recycled to cell membrane or to the trans-Golgi network [29].

3.3. Binding and regulation of IGF2 mitogenic effects

M6P/IGF2-R binds to IGF2 with higher affinity, Kd = 0.1–1 nM [37, 38] and has a lower affinity for IGF1 [39]. By contrast, it does not bind to insulin [40].

The mitogenic effects of IGF2 are exerted by its binding with lower affinity to the signaling receptors such as the IGF1 receptor or insulin receptor isoform A [9]. M6P/IGF2-R acts as a scavenger by mediating internalization and degradation of IGF2 as described previously in cell cultures including rat adipocytes [41] mouse L-cells [42]. In vivo, studies provide evidence that M6P/IGF2-R regulates IGF2 circulating and tissue amounts, as shown by gene deletion experiments in mice [43, 44]. These studies reported that in mice-deficient M6P/IGF2-R, IGF2 levels were two- to threefold increased than wild type. Moreover, the lack of M6P/IGF2-R increased levels and induces tissue proliferation and hypertrophy that is produced by IGF2 acting on the IGF1 receptor [45].

3.4. Binding to mannose-6-phosphorylated molecules

3.4.1. Transforming growth factor β1

The M6P/IGF2-R is involved in proteolytic activation of the transforming growth factor β1 (TGFβ1), a potent growth inhibitor, that regulates the differentiation and growth in most cell types [46]. *TGFβ1* is a mannose-6-phosphorylated protein synthesized as a single inactive propreprotein, which is secreted and stored in extracellular matrix. Inactive *TGFβ* binds to M6P/IGF2-R and it is then cleaved in mature and active form by extracellular plasmin [47]. This activation mechanism of *TGFβ* by M6P/IGF2-R has been described in cell culture model but not in vivo [46, 30]. Moreover, several studies suggested a role of plasmin-mediated activation of inactive *TGFβ* following its binding to the M6P/IGF2-R [46, 48, 49].

M6P/IGF2-R is known to bind to domains DII and DII of urokinase receptor [50]. So, other studies suggest the binding of plasminogen to the complex M6P/IGF2-R/urokinase plasminogen activator receptor, leading to the generation of active plasmin that activates receptor-bound latent *TGFβ* [51, 52].

3.4.2. Retinoic acid

Retinoic acid plays an important role in development, cellular metabolism, and regulation of cell proliferation. The retinoic acid binds to a specific signaling nuclear receptor. Kang et al. [53] reported that the retinoic acid binds to the cytoplasmic domain of M6P/IGF2-R. Retinoic acid has been shown to stimulate M6P/IGF2 receptor-mediated internalization of IGF2 and to increase lysosomal enzymes sorting [30]. M6P/IGF2-R has been proposed to play a role in mediating retinoid-induced apoptosis/growth inhibition [29].

3.4.3. Leukemia inhibitory factor

M6P/IGF2-R is involved in the internalization and degradation of the cytokine leukemia inhibitory factor (LIF) leading to its regulation [54].

http://dx.doi.org/10.5772/64810

3.4.4. Proliferin

Proliferin is a paracrine factor related to prolactin glycoprotein involved in endothelial cells, angiogenesis during fetal development [55, 56], and a mitogen-regulated protein previously described in mouse 3T3 fibroblasts [57, 58]. Its signaling pathway suggests a G protein-coupled receptor [59] but remains unclear.

3.4.5. Prorenin

The prorenin is a proenzyme secreted by juxtaglomerular cells of kidney. The renin catalyzes the activation of angiotensin I into angiotensin II that regulates blood pressure and extracellular fluid volume [60]. Mannose-6-phosphorylated prorenin [61] binding to M6P/IGF2-R leads to its internalization and proteolytic activation into renin.

3.4.6. Thyroglobulin

Studies showed that radiolabeled thyroglobulin binds to M6P/IGF2-R [62]. Moreover, thyroglobulin can be endocytosed by the M6P/IGF2-R but the receptor fails to direct it to the lysosomes for its degradation in the thyroid gland [63].

4. Does the M6P/IGF2-R interact with G-proteins?

The function of M6P/IGF2-R as a signaling receptor is poorly understood and controversial. Several studies reported that M6P/IGF2-R lacks intrinsic kinase activity, contrarily to insulin and IGF1 receptors. The authors suggested that M6P/IGF2-R is coupled to G-protein via a 14-amino acids sequence (^{2410}RVGLVRGEKARKGK^{2423}) localized in the cytoplasmic domain of the M6P/IGF2-R (**Figure 1**) that is similar to the third cytoplasmic loop of G-protein-coupled seven transmembrane region receptors [64]. Nishimoto et al. [65] showed that IGF2 binds to M6P/IGF2-R and stimulated calcium channel in mouse Balb/c3T3 cells. Moreover this action of IGF2 on calcium influx was abolished by *Bordetella pertussis* toxin or by using antibodies directed against M6P/IGF2-R, suggesting a G protein-mediated biological effect of M6P/IGF2-R [66]. By contrast, others showed that mice L-cells expressing wild or mutated M6P/IGF2-R and treated to *B. pertussis* toxin were capable to block toxin-inhibiting activity. These last results showed an absence of coupling between M6P/IGF2-R and G-protein [67]. Recent studies using HEK293 cells suggested a novel mechanism of IGF2-mediated G-protein activation. In that model, IGF2 binding to M6P/IGF2-R leads to activation of sphingosine kinase and production of extracellular sphingosine 1-phosphate (S1P), the ligand for G protein-coupled S1P receptors [68]. Others suggested that mannose-6-phosphorylated ligands of M6P/IGF2-R also used that pathway [59]. However, there is no direct evidence involving the binding of these ligands and sphingosine kinase activation. Most of biological effects of IGF2 are mediated by IGF1 receptor and insulin receptor [30]. This pathway probably occurs in chicken since IGF2 stimulates protein synthesis and fibroblast mitosis in that species, whereas mannose-6-phosphate receptor does not bind to IGF2 [15].

5. Role in human cancers

The study of M6P/IGF2-R in the targeting of newly synthesized mannose-6-phosphorylated lysosomal enzymes, such as cathepsin D, in human breast cancer lines showed that pro-cathepsin D is secreted from cancer cell lines, suggesting a possible alteration of M6P/IGF2-R [69].

Studies on M6P/IGF2-R gene localized on 6q chromosome (6q25–27 region) in human mammary cancers showed losses of heterozygosity (LOH) in 48% of tumors [70, 71].

Further studies showed that M6P/IGF2-R gene exhibited LOH in 30% of breast cancer with informative mutations in 2/5 of the remaining allele [72]. The LOH phenomenon has been confirmed in mammary cancers [73] and also described in other human cancers such as hepatocarcinoma [74] and ovarian cancers [75]. Studies at the protein level in mammary cancer showed that M6P/IGF2-R levels were significantly lower in cancer cells than in normal cells in 50% of tumors in which the peritumoral normal glands could be quantified in parallel, agreeing the hypothesis of a tumor suppressor gene for the M6P/IGF2-R [76]. Most of further studies led on M6P/IGF2-R suggested M6P/IGF2-R as being coded by a tumor suppressor gene [72, 77, 78] and its role as a putative prognostic marker in breast cancers has been hypothesized [76].

6. Conclusion

The M6P/IGF2-R is a multifunctional receptor that is known as binding molecules sharing M6P signals and IGF2. Further studies showed that it also binds to many other mannose-6-phosphorylated molecules such as TGFβ, retinoic acid, and so on. The M6P/IGF2-R is a single-chain membrane receptor consisting of a large extracellular domain of 2264 amino acids residues organized in 15 repeats, a short transmembrane of 23 amino acids residues, and a small intracellular domain of 164 residues. The receptor targets newly synthesized mannose-6-phosphorylated lysosomal enzymes by binding M6P signals on specific sites localized in repeats 3 and 9 of extracellular domain and transports them from the trans-Golgi network to lysosomal compartment. The secreted enzymes precursors are internalized by the M6P/IGF2-R localized on the cell membrane and routed to lysosomes for their maturation. IGF2 binds to repeat 11 of the receptor and is transported, after internalization, to the lysosomes for its degradation. IGF2 effects on growth and development are mediated by IGF1 or insulin receptors, although these receptors bind IGF2 with lower affinity. Consequently, M6P/IGF2-R is considered as a scavenger that regulates IGF2 levels before it reaches IGF1 receptor to exert its biological effects on cell proliferation and growth. M6P/IGF2-R would be considered as a "Garbage Receptor," since it does not lead to a known biochemical pathway of signal transduction but transports its ligands to lysosomes for degradation, in opposition to "Signaling Receptor" that induces signal transduction after ligand binding.

The M6P/IGF2-R gene maps on chromosome 6q region and is imprinted in rodents, whereas its expression is mostly biallelic in human. M6P/IGF2-R gene has been suggested as acting as a tumor suppressor since losses of heterozygosity and mutations in the remaining allele have been frequently described in many human tumors such as mammary, ovarian, and liver cancers. These previous results are supported by the measures of M6P/IGF2-R at the protein level showing significant decrease of receptor levels in cancer cells than in normal cells in about 50% of breast tumors, which led to suggest its potential value as a cancer prognostic marker.

Insulin-like growth factor axis has a critical role in mediating fetal and postnatal growth; thus, alterations in this pathway including changes in the expression of the M6P/IGF2-receptor and impairments in its function could impact somatic growth. Moreover, genetic evidence clearly supports a role for IGF2/M6P receptors in organ development and growth.

Author details

Guy Joseph Lemamy[1,2*], Bénédicte Ndeboko[2], Serge Thierry Omouessi[2] and Justine Mouecoucou[2]

*Address all correspondence to: guylemamy@yahoo.fr

1 National Institute of Health and Medical Research (INSERM) U148, Montpellier, France

2 University of Health Sciences, Faculty of Medicine, Libreville, Gabon

References

[1] Morgan D.O., Edman J.C., Standring D.N., Fried V.A., Smith M.C., Roth R.A., Rutter W.J. Insulin-like growth factor II receptor as a multifunctional binding protein. Nature 1987; 329: 301–307.

[2] MacDonald R.G., Pfeffer S.R., Coussens L., Tepper M.A., Brocklebank C.M., Mole J.E., Anderson J.K., Chen E., Czech M.P., Ullrich A. A Single Receptor binds both Insulin-like Growth Factor 2 and Mannose-6-Phosphate. Science 1988; 239: 1134–1137.

[3] Hoflack B., Kornfeld D. Purification and characterization of a cation-dependent mannose-6-phosphate receptor from murine P388D1 macrophages and bovine liver. J Biol Chem 1995; 260: 12008–12014.

[4] Salmon W.D.J., Daughaday W.H. A hormonally controlled serum factor which stimulates sulphate incorporation by cartilage in vitro. J Lab Clin Med 1957; 49: 825–836.

[5] Rinderknecht E., Humbel R.E. The amino acid sequence of human insulin-like growth factor I and its structural homology with pro-Insulin. J Biol Chem 1978; 253: 2769–2776.

[6] Rinderknecht E., Humbel R.E. Primary structure of insulin-like growth factor II. FEBS Lett 1978; 89: 283–286.

[7] Engström W., Shokrai A., Otte K., Granérus M., Gessbo A., Bierke P., Madej A., Sjölund M., Ward A. Transcriptional regulation and biological significance of insulin-like growth factor II gene. Cell Prolif 1998; 31: 173–189.

[8] Zumkeller W. IGFs and IGFBPs: surrogate markers for diagnosis and surveillance of tumor growth. J Clin Pathol Mol Pathol 2001; 54: 285–288.

[9] Bergman D., Halje M., Nordin M., Engström W. Insulin-like growth factor 2 in development and disease: a mini-review. Gerontology 2013; 59: 240–249.

[10] Gamroudi F., Mac Donald R.G. Localization of the insulin-like growth factor ii (IGFII) binding/cross-linking site of the IGFII mannose-6-phosphate receptor to extracellular 10–11. J Biol Chem 1994; 269: 26944–26952.

[11] Hancock M.K., Haskins D.J., Sun G., Dahms N.M. Identification of residues essential for carbohydrate recognition by the insulin-like growth factor II/mannose-6-phosphate receptor. J Biol Chem 2002; 277 (13): 11255–11264.

[12] Hassan A.B. Keys to the hidden treasures of the mannose-6-phosphate/insulin-like growth factor 2 receptor. Am J Pathol 2003; 162: 3–6.

[13] Hancock M.K., Yammani R.D., Dahms N.M. Localization of the carbohydrate recognition sites of the insulin-like growth factor ii/mannose-6-phosphate receptor to domains 3 and 9 of the extracytoplasmic region. J Biol Chem 2002; 277 (49): 47205–47212.

[14] Schmidt B., Kiecke-Siemsen C., Waheed A., Braulke T., Von Figura K. Localization of the insulin-like growth factor II binding site to the amino-acids 1508-1566 in repeat 11of the mannose-6-phosphate/insulin-like growth factor II receptor. J Biol Chem 1995; 270: 14975–14982.

[15] Clairmont K.B., Czech M.P. Chicken and xenopus mannose-6-phosphate receptors fail to bind insulin-like growth factor II. J Biol Chem 1989; 264: 16390–16392.

[16] Confort C., Rochefort H., Vignon F. Insulin-like growth factors (IGFs) stimulate the release of α_2-antichymotrypsin and soluble IGFII/mannose-6-phosphate receptor from MCF7 breast cancer cells. Endocrinology 1995; 136: 3759–3766.

[17] Kiess W., Greenstein L.A., White R.M., Lee L., Rechler M.M., Nissley S.P. Type II insulin-like growth factor receptor is present in rat serum. Proc Natl Acad Sci USA 1987; 84: 7720–7724.

[18] Causin C., Waheed A., Braulke T., Junghans U., Maly P., Humbel R.E., Von Figura K. Mannose-6-posphate/Insulin-like growth factor II binding proteins in human serum and urine. Their relation to the mannose-6-posphate/insulin-like growth factor II receptor. Biochem J 1988; 252: 795–799.

[19] MacDonald R.G., Tepper M.A., Clairmont K.B., Perregaux S.B., Czech M.P. Serum form of the rat insulin-like growth factor II/mannose-6-phosphate receptor is truncated in the carboxyl-terminal domain. J Biol Chem 1989; 264 (6): 3256–3261.

[20] Laureys G., Barton D.E., Ullrich A., Francke U. Chromosomal mapping of the gene for the type II insulin-like growth factor/cation independent mannose-6-phosphate receptor in man and mouse. Genomics 1988; 3: 224–229.

[21] Szebenyi G., Rotwein P. The mouse insulin-like growth factor II/cation independent mannose-6-phosphate (OGFII/MPR) receptor gene: molecular cloning and genomic organization. Genomics 1994; 19: 120–129.

[22] Brown J., Jones E., Forbes B.E. Interaction of IGFII with the IGF-2R/cation independent mannose-6-phosphate receptor mechanism and biological outcomes Vitam Horm 2009; 80: 699–719.

[23] Ward A. Beckwith-Wiedemann syndrome and Wilms' tumor. Mol Hum Reprod 1997; 3: 157–168.

[24] Kalscheuer V.M., Mariman E.C., Scheppens M.T., Rehder H., Ropens H.H. The insulin-like growth factor type 2 receptor is imprinted in mouse but not in humans. Nat Gent 1993; 5: 74–78.

[25] Killian J.K., Nolan C.M., Wylie A.A., Li T., Vu T.H., Hoffman A.R., Jirtle R.L. Divergent evolution in M6P/IGF2R imprinting from the Jurassic to the Quaternary. Human Mol Genet 2001; 10: 1721–1728.

[26] Abu-Amero S., Monk D., Apostolidou S., Stanier P., Moore G. Imprinted genes and their role in human fetal growth. Cytogenet Genome Res 2006; 113: 262–270.

[27] Natowicz M., Hallet D.W., Frier C., Chi M., Schesinger P.H., Barenziger J.U. Recognition and receptor-mediated uptake of phosphorylated high mannose-type oligosaccharides by cultured human fibroblasts. J Cell Biol 1983; 96: 915–919.

[28] Tong P.Y., Gregory W., Kornfeld S. Ligands interactions of the cation-independent mannose-6-phoshate receptor. J Biol Chem 1989; 264: 7962–7969.

[29] Dahms N.M., Lobel P., Kornfeld S. Mannose-6-phosphate receptors and lysosomal enzymes targeting. J Biol Chem 1989; 264: 12115–12118.

[30] Kornfeld S. Structure and function of the mannose-6-phosphate/insulin-like growth factor II receptor. Ann Rev Biochem 1992; 61: 307–330.

[31] Von Figura K., Hasilik A. Lysosomal enzymes and their receptors. Ann Rev Biochem 1986; 55: 167–193.

[32] Chen H.J., Remmler J., Delaney J.C., Messner D.J., Lobel P. Mutational analysis of the cation-independent mannose-6-phosphate/insulin-like growth factor II receptor. J Biol Chem 1993; 268: 22336–22346.

[33] Sandoval I.V., Bakke O. Targeting of membrane proteins to endosomes and lysosomes. Trends Cell Biol 1994; 4: 292–297.

[34] Oka Y., Czech M.P. The type II insulin-like growth factor is internalized and recycled in the absence of ligand. J Biol Chem 1986; 261: 9090–9093.

[35] Lobel P., Fujimoto K., Griffiths G., Kornfeld S. Mutations in cytoplasmic domain the 275 kDa mannose-6-phosphate receptor differentially alter lysosomal enzymes sorting and endocytosis. Cell 1989; 57: 787–796.

[36] Jadot M., Canfield M.M., Gregory W., Kornfeld S. Characterization of the signal for rapid internalization of the bovine mannose-6-phosphate/insulin-like growth factor II receptor. J Biol Chem 1992; 267: 11069–11077.

[37] Oppenheimer C.L., Czech M.P. Purification of the type II insulin-like growth factor receptor from rat placenta. J Biol Chem 1983; 258: 8539–8542.

[38] August G.P., Nissley S.P., Kasuga M., Lee L., Greenstein L., Rechler M.M. Purification of insulin-like growth factor II receptor from rat chondosarcoma cells. J Biol Chem 1983; 258: 9033–9036.

[39] Nissley S.P., and Kiess W. Binding of Insulin-like Growth Factor II (IGFII) and Lysosomal Enzymes to the IGFII/Mannose-6-Phosphate Receptor. In Modern Concepts of Insulin- like Growth Factors. Spencer E.M. (ed.). New York; Elsevier Science Publishing 1991: 419–430.

[40] Rosenfeld R.G., Conover C.A., Hodges D., Lee P.D., Misra P., Hintz R.L., Li C.H. Heterogeneity of insulin-like growth factor I affinity for the insulin-like growth factor II receptor comparison of natural, synthetic and recombinant cDNA-derived insulin-like growth factor I. Biochem Biophys Res Comm 1987; 143: 199–205.

[41] Oka Y., Rozek I.M., Czech M.P. Direct demonstration of rapid insulin-like growth factor II receptor internalization and recycling in rat adipocytes. Insulin stimulates 125I-insulin-like growth factor II degradation by modulating the IGF-II receptor recycling process. J Biol Chem 1985; 260: 9435–9442.

[42] Nolan C.M., Kyle J.W., Watanabe H., Sly W.S. Binding of insulin-like growth factor II by human cation-independent mannose-6-phosphate/IGFII receptor expressed in receptor deficient mouse L-cells. Cell Regul 1990; 1: 197–213.

[43] Ludwig T., Eggenschwier J., Fisher P., D'Ercole A.J., Davenport M.L., Efstratiadis A. Mouse mutants lacking the type 2 IGF receptor (IGF2R) are rescued from perinatal lethality in IGF2 and IGF2R null backgrounds. Dev Biol 1996; 177: 517–535.

[44] Wang Z.Q., Fung M.R., Barlow D.P., Wagner E.F. Regulation of embryonic growth and lysosomal targeting by the imprinted IGF2/MPR gene. Nature 1994; 372: 464–467.

[45] Lau M.M., Stewart C.E., Liu Z., Bhatt H., Rotwein P., Stewart C.L. Loss of the imprinted IGF2/cation-independent mannose-6-phosphate receptor results in fetal overgrowth and perinatal lethality. Genes Dev 1994; 8: 2953–2963.

[46] Dennis P.A., Rifkin D.B. Cellular activation of latent transforming growth inhibitor β requires binding to the cation-independent mannosr-6-phosphate/insulin-like growth factor type II receptor. Proc Natl Acad Sci USA 1991; 88: 580–584.

[47] Flaumenhaft R., Kojima S., Abe M., Rifkin D.B. Activation of latent transforming factor beta. Adv Pharmacol 1993; 24: 51–76.

[48] Ghahary A., Tredget E.E., Mi L., Yang L. Cellular response to latent TGF beta1 is facilitate by insulin-like growth factor II/mannose-6-phosphate receptors on MS-9 cells. Exp Cell Res 1999; 25: 111–120.

[49] Villevalois-Le-Cam L., Rescan C., Gilot D., Ezan F., Loyer P., Desbuquois B., Guguen-Guillouzo C., Baffet G. The hepatocyte is a direct target for transforming growth factor beta activation via insulin-like growth factor II/mannose-6-phosphate receptor. J Hepatol 2003; 38: 156–163.

[50] Nykjaer A., Christensen E.I., Vorum H., Hager H., Petersen C.M., Roigaard H., Min H.Y., Vilhardt F., Moller L.B., Kornfeld S., Gliemann J. Mannose-6-phosphate/insulin-like growth factor 2 receptor targets the urokinase receptor to lysosomes via a novel binding interaction. J Cell Biol 1998; 141: 815–828.

[51] Godar S., Horejsi V., Weidle U.H., Binder B.R., Hansmann C., Stockinger H. M6P/IGFII receptor complexes urokinase receptor and plasminogen for activation of transforming growth factor-beta1. Eur J Immunol 1999; 29: 1004–1013.

[52] Kreiling J.L., Byrd J.C., Deisz R.J., Mizukami I.F., Todd R.F.I., MacDonald R.G. Binding of urokinase-type plasminogen activator receptor (uPAR) to the mannose-6-phosphate/insulin-like growth factor II receptor: contrasting interaction of full-length an soluble forms of uPAR. J Biol Chem 2003; 278: 20628–20637.

[53] Kang J.X., Li Y., Leaf A. Mannose-6-phosphate/insulin-like growth factor 2 receptor is a receptor for retinoic acid. Proc Natl Acad Sci USA 1998; 95: 13671–13676.

[54] Blanchard F., Duplomb L., Raher S., Vusio P., Hoflack B., Jacques Y., Godard A. Mannose-6-phosphate/insulin-like growth factor II receptor mediates internalization and degradation of leukemia inhibitory factor but not signal transduction. J Biol Chem 1999; 274: 24685–24693.

[55] Linzer D.I., Nathans D. Nucleotide sequence of a growth-related mRNA encoding a member of the prolactin-growth hormone family. Proc Natl Acad Sci USA 1984; 81: 4255–4259.

[56] Nilsen-Hamilton M., Shapiro J.M., Massoglia S.L., Hamilton R.T. Selective stimulations by mitogens of incorporation of35S-methionine into a family of proteins released into the medium by 3T3 cells. Cell 1980; 20: 19–28.

[57] Lee S.J., Nathans D. Proliferin secreted by cultured cells binds to mannose-6-phosphate receptors. J Biol Chem 1988; 263: 3521–3527.

[58] Linzer D.I., Nathans D. A new member of the prolactin-growth hormone gene family expressed in mouse placenta. EMBO J 1985; 4: 1419–1423.

[59] Groskopf J.C., Syu L.J., Saltiel A.R., Linzer D.I. Proliferin induces endothelial chemotaxis through a G protein-coupled, mitogen-activated protein kinase-dependent pathway. Endocrinology 1997; 138: 2835–2840.

[60] Lacasse J., Ballak M., Mercure C., Gutkowsska J., Chapeau C., Foote S., Menard J., Corvol P., Cantin M., Genest J. Immunohistochemical localization of renin in juxtaglomerular cells. J Histochem Cytochem 1985; 33: 323–332.

[61] Faust P.L., Chirgwin J.M., Kornfeld S. Renin, a secretory glycoprotein, acquires phosphomannosyl residues. J Cell Biol 1987; 105: 1947–1955.

[62] Herzog V., Neumüller W., Holzmann B. Thyroglobulin, the major and obligatory exportable protein of thyroid follicle cells, carries the lysosomal recognition marker mannose-6-phosphate. EMBO J 1987; 6: 555–560.

[63] Lemansky P., Herzog V. Endocytosis of thyroglobulin is not mediated by mannose-6-phosphate receptors in thyrocytes. Evidence for low-affinity-binding sites operating in the uptake of thyroglobulin. Eur J Biochem 1992; 209:111–119.

[64] Okamoto T., Katada T., Murayama Y., Ui M., Ogata E., Nishimoto I. A simple structure encodes G-protein activating function of the IGFII/mannose-6-phosphate receptor. Cell 1990; 62: 709–717.

[65] Nishimoto I., Hata Y., Ogata E., Kojima I. Insulin-like growth factor II stimulates calcium influx in competent Balbc/3T3 cells primed with epidermal growth factor. J Biol Chem 1987; 262: 12120–12126.

[66] Nishimoto I., Murayama Y., Katada T., Ui M., Ogata E. Possible direct linkage of insulin-like growth factor II receptor with guanine nucleotide-binding proteins. J Biol Chem 1989; 264: 14029–14038.

[67] Körner C., Nürnberg B., Uhde M., Braulke T. Mannose-6-phosphate/insulin-like growth factor II receptor fails to interact with G-proteins. J Biol Chem 1995; 270: 287–295.

[68] El-Shewy H.M., Johnson K.R., Lee M.H., Jaffa A.A., Obeid L.M., Luttrell L.M. Insulin-like growth factors mediate heterotrimeric G protein-dependent ERK1/2 activation by transactivating sphingosine 1-phosphate receptors. J Biol Chem 2006; 281: 31399–31407.

[69] Westley B., Rochefort H. A secreted glycoprotein induced by estrogen in human breast cancer lines. Cell 1980; 20: 352–362.

[70] Sheng Z.M., Marchetti A., Buttitta F., Champeme M.H., Campani D., Bistocchi M., Lidereau R., Callahan R. Multiple regions of chromosome 6q affected by loss of heterozygosity in primary breast carcinomas. Br J Cancer 1996; 73: 144–147.

[71] Noviello C., Courjal F., Theillet C. Loss of heterozygosity on the long arm of chromosome 6 in breast cancer: possibly four regions of deletions. Clin Cancer Res 1996; 2: 1601–1606.

[72] Hankins G.R., De Souza A.T., Bentley R.C., Patel M.R., Marks J.R., Iglehart J.D., Jirtle R.L. M6P/IGF2 receptor: a candidate breast tumor suppressor gene. Oncogene 1996; 12: 2003–2009.

[73] Chapell S.A., Walsh T., Walker R.A., Shaw J.A. Loss of heterozygosity at the mannose-6-phosphate/insulin-like growth factor 2 receptor gene correlates with poor differentiation in early breast carcinoma. Br J Cancer 1997; 76: 1558–1561.

[74] De Souza A.T., Hankins G.R., Washington M.K., Fine L.F., Orton T.C., Jirtle R.L. Frequent loss of heterozygosity on 6q at the mannose-6-phosphate/insulin-like growth factor II receptor locus in human hepatocellular tumors. Oncogene 1995; 10: 1725–1729.

[75] Saïto S., Sirahama S., Matsushima M., Suzuki M., Sagae S., Kudo R., Saito J., Noda K., Nakumura Y. Definition of commonly deleted region in ovarian cancer to 300-kb segment of chromosome 6q27. Cancer Res 1996; 56: 5586–5589.

[76] Lemamy G.J., Roger P., Mani J.C., Berthe M.L., Rochefort H., Brouillet J.P. High affinity antibodies from hen's egg yolk against human mannose-6-phosphate/insulin-like growth factor 2 receptor (M6P/IGF2-R): characterization and potential use in clinical cancer studies. Int J Cancer 1999; 80: 896–902.

[77] Oates A.J., Schumaker L.M., Jenkins S.B., Pearce A.A., DaCosta S.A., Arun B., Ellis M.J.C. The mannose-6-phosphate/insulin-like growth factor 2 receptor (M6P/IGF2R), a putative breast tumor suppressor gene. Breast Cancer Res Treat 1998; 47: 269–281.

[78] Lemamy G.J., Esslimani Sahla M., Berthe M.L., Roger P. Is the mannose-6-phosphate/insulin-like growth factor 2 receptor coded by a breast cancer suppressor gene? Adv Exp Med Biol 2008; 617: 305–310.